RACING FOR A MIRACLE

MIRACLE

RONNIE'S CANCER JOURNEY

RONNIE CAMPBELL

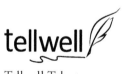

Tellwell Talent
www.tellwell.ca

ISBN
978-0-2288-5373-2 (Hardcover)
978-0-2288-5372-5 (Paperback)
978-0-2288-5374-9 (eBook)

TABLE OF CONTENTS

Diagnosis: Aggressive Stage 4 colon cancer

Definition of colon cancer:

"Cancer is considered suppressed rage; when cancer is part of our digestive system, it is an indicator that there is something we are having trouble releasing." (Louise Hay)

I am not always brave. But I am here, and in the moment, focused on being grateful, grounded, centered, and positive.

I am feeling the blessings and the gift of God's love and his power. I am living proof of a miracle he has bestowed on me throughout my cancer journey.

My hope is you are open to reading my story. You will not feel alone on your personal journey because I will share my reality and my truths. Through my eyes, may you experience my struggles and my celebrations.

-

PART 1

The Diagnosis 2018

I remember that day like it was yesterday.

May 24, 2018

I t was the day my life changed forever. I left work for a follow-up on my colonoscopy. I was the last patient of the day. The doctor says hello, and opens my file to go over the results. He starts by saying they had found what looks like a cancerous tumour. I have surgery scheduled to remove the tumour. My doctor then goes over to a diagram on the wall and says, we will cut here and here, ensuring the cancer is removed. First, though, I have a scheduled CAT scan tomorrow. The surgery is scheduled in two weeks. At this point, I don't remember anything else he said. I felt numb.

I thought to myself: *Am I hearing him correctly? Is this for real? It can't be. I am healthy and fit. I am never sick.* I came to the doctor's thinking the usual—everything is normal. I am good to go. See you in five years.

Not today. I left the examining room. I start to leave for the office, and the nurse calls me back. "Veronica, here are papers and information you need for your upcoming appointments."

I am still thinking to myself: *this can't be real.* I walked to my car, sat for a moment, then said, "What the Fuck Just Happened in there? How could I have cancer?"

I remember calling my husband to let him know. He couldn't believe it. Once home, I looked over the information regarding my CAT scan and surgery while waiting for my son to come home so I could tell him. I had a CAT scan scheduled for the next day. I had never had a CAT scan before or even major surgery. My labor and delivery with my son were considered easy. Still trying to take it all in, I called my boss to let him know I would be off tomorrow. I told him the doctor wanted to run some more tests, and I would be back on Monday.

I still could not believe surgery was in two weeks. We were stunned by the news and wondered why everything had been scheduled so quickly. Could it be really bad? Or was this just the way cancer was treated? All I knew is that I had no time to think. I tried to remain positive that the tumour would be removed, and I'd be back to work in six weeks. Great! Thank God! I would have the summer off. My mind raced, thinking this has to be early-stage cancer since I just had a colonoscopy sixteen months earlier in Tennessee. Had the doctor in Tennessee missed something? Could the tumour have been there all this time?

I want to go back to January 2017 to put all this in context. I was living and working in Tennessee at the time. It was near the end of my two-year work term. In December 2016, my identical twin was diagnosed with breast cancer. Being identical twins, I wanted to be safe and get the tests required as a precautionary measure to confirm I, too, did not have any cancer. I scheduled appointments for a mammogram, Pap smear, and colonoscopy.

My appointments were scheduled for January 2017. My mammogram and Pap smear came back normal, but the colonoscopy did not. The doctor said she was unable to complete the exam. She had removed some precancerous pulps and recommended I get another colonoscopy in six months. Since I was moving back home to Canada in May 2017, I thought I would just schedule and redo all of the tests once back in Canada with my family doctor. In June 2017, I met with my family doctor so she could schedule the appointments. I mentioned the recommendation to have another colonoscopy within six months since the doctor in Tennessee was unable to complete the exam. Then I gave my family doctor all of the medical reports with my results from the examinations in Tennessee.

My mammogram and Pap smear were scheduled immediately, but my colonoscopy was not. Time went by. I had started a new job, and my family doctor retired. I had a new family doctor who had reviewed my file. It had been so long since I had requested the appointment. I actually forgot about my request. In hindsight, would things have been different if it had been done in June of 2017? We will never know.

May 25, 2018

I go for my first CAT scan—as I would soon learn, it would be one of many. When I get there, the nurse asks me what kind of juice I want. I say apple. With a CAT scan, you need to drink two large glasses of 'oral contrast'— a liquid that contains barium. I drink and wait an hour for it to go through my system. Then, I go to the imaging room where the CAT scan would be done.

CAT scan. You lie in a tunnel-like machine while the inside of the machine rotates and takes a series of X-rays from different angles. These pictures are then sent to a computer, where they're combined to create images of slices, or cross-sections, of the body.

Doctors order CAT scans for a long list of reasons:

They can help locate a tumour, blood clot, excess fluid, or infection. Doctors use them to guide treatment plans and procedures, such as biopsies, surgeries, and radiation therapy.

Doctors can compare CAT scans to find out if certain treatments are working. For example, scans of a tumour over time can show whether the body is responding to the chemo or radiation in a manner it was intended.

The technician hooked up an IV. He tells me when they inject the liquid, it will feel like you have wet your pants. The scan starts, and he announces, "I am going to do the injection," and oh my God, I thought I had peed my pants. It was so weird. I was afraid to get off the table. The CAT scan itself takes about ten minutes.

The weekend was a blur, and then Monday, I was back at work. I explained to my boss what was happening. I had surgery scheduled in two weeks. Hopefully, everything would go well, and I would back at work in six weeks. The more I thought about what was happening, the more my gut was saying, "Maybe there was something on the report and I missed it" I took out the Tennessee medical reports to look at them again. I wanted to review the results and look at the pictures. I was not sure what I was looking for—had I waited too long?

June 13, 2018

My surgery day. I hardly slept last night. I am so nervous about what will happen today. Yesterday I cycled sixty kilometres, thinking it may be a while before I can do this again. I will get one more ride in while I am healthy. I just kept thinking to myself: I have zero symptoms; I feel great. Maybe I have nothing to worry about? It will just be a normal surgery to remove the tumour, and I'll heal and be back at work in six weeks.

I arrive at the hospital at 6:00 a.m. The medical team set up my IV and start pre-meds for surgery. I'm still feeling pretty good and wondering what I am doing there, but deep down, I had a gut feeling things would not be good.

They start to wheel me to the operating room. I give my husband, Dave, a kiss, and off I go. In the operating room, the anaesthetist asks me to sit up on the table, lean forward, and he injects my lower back with pain meds. The next thing I remember is waking up in recovery with a sore abdomen. When I glanced down, it looked like a turtle shell on my stomach—protection for my incision area. My incision went from under my bra line to the top of my pelvic bone, and there were fifty staples. In the recovery room, Dave and my son Curtis and his friend were waiting for me. The doctor came in. He went over the surgery and his findings. He said they removed about twelve and a half inches of my intestines, scraped my lymph nodes, and to his surprise, there was another satellite tumour on my stomach cavity on the omentum, which he removed. This tumour did not show on the CAT scan I had had two weeks ago. Everything was removed and sent to be tested for cancer.

I was tired and in a lot of discomfort. I could barely stay awake, so my family did not stay long. I do remember later during the night, a nurse asking me to try and get out of the bed. She needed to be sure I could move. I was not sure how I was going to do that without splitting in half. It was so painful to stand up. My core muscles were so sore. I had a very restless night with little sleep as I could not get comfortable. Being a side sleeper, I now had to sleep on my back. I spent four days in the hospital. My son visited me daily, bringing me a green tea and saying, "Mom, you need to get up, walk down the hall and do steps so you can come home." I could barely sit up, let alone get out of bed to walk steps. My son, twenty-eight, had never seen me sick.

He was used to his mom being active and always on the go, so for him to experience his mom lying in a hospital bed was very strange.

Day Five. I was excited to be going home. The doctor arrived to release me. He told me I had an appointment scheduled for next week to remove my staples and review my surgery results.

He left, and the nurse checked my incision and changed my dressing. She spent time going over how to care for my incision, and I was finally ready to go home.

The drive home was not easy. I did not realize how much it hurt to sit and how low my seat was in my car. I had been lying or standing only for the last five days. Bending was a different story. My husband reclined my seat as far as it would go, and I put my hands under my buttocks to buffer the bumps. Thank goodness we live close to the hospital. I was so glad to be home. The very first thing I did was take a shower. After the shower, I felt better than I had in days. I continued to struggle with sitting, and I found standing was more comfortable. Sleeping was another struggle— trying to find my comfortable position.

June 21, 2018

Today was the visit to the surgeon's office to review my results. I will have half of the fifty staples removed from my abdominal area. The surgeon explained he had removed twelve and a half inches of my intestine around the tumour area. He said for a small woman, I had a lot of intestines. He removed thirty lymph nodes—two were positive for cancer. The surprise tumour on my omentum also tested positive for cancer. He explains I will now have to undergo chemotherapy treatments. He had already set up an appointment with an oncologist at the cancer clinic. He informs me the oncologist will meet with me to discuss the cancer and my chemo treatments. It was not the result we had hoped for. I am feeling frightened but will get through it. I text updates to all of our family to let them know the outcome.

June 27, 2018

I ventured out for a little walk in the morning. I knew it would not be a long walk, but it would be a change from walking around the pool. In the afternoon, I was back to the surgeon's office to have the remaining staples removed. I found it a little tender at the belly button. I am nervous about the next appointment later today with my oncologist. I do not want to be sick and lose my hair as my sister did. Hopefully, we will find out the start date of chemo and how many sessions I will need. Dave and I were both nervous when we arrived at the cancer clinic. The nurse came into the examining room first. She introduced herself, handed me a little bag with some chemotherapy, chemo port/chemo PICC information, and a pair of socks. I am sure the nurse was trying to make us feel comfortable and not overwhelmed and frightened. She told me she would be my contact at the cancer clinic if I have questions or if anything is wrong.

Then the oncologist came into the room to introduce himself and started to review the surgery results. He commented on how well I looked for someone who had recently had surgery. Then Dave asked, "before you go on, can we record this?" The oncologist said certainly; then he went on to tell us the colon cancer had been removed, along with the local lymph nodes, and that this was standard procedure. The surprise from the surgery was the satellite tumour on the omentum that covers all the abdominal organs. He informed us when cancer spreads outside of the tumour area; it is considered Stage 4 cancer. Also, Stage 4 is treated very differently than other stages of cancer since it is the final stage.

He assures us that even though we had a great surgeon, there is still a very high chance I still have cancer in my body. It has already spread to the omentum, so it has likely spread to other organs in my abdominal area. I could not believe what I was hearing.

He suggested I have another scan of my whole body to ensure that cancer has not spread to other organs. He then talks to us about the chemo, saying that the chemo I will have will never clear the cancer. What it will do is help to slow down the cancer's spread. Either way, it is not looking good. He looks at Dave and me and says he recommends two possible treatment options. Since I was young and healthy, the first option would be his choice if my CAT scan results showed the cancer had not spread to the other organs.

Option number one. You are a perfect candidate for a surgery called HIPEC, he told me. This surgery is supposed to work better than normal chemo for this type of cancer. This procedure is done by opening up the stomach, checking all of the organs to ensure no cancer, then inserting two probes that will allow warm chemo at a temperature of forty-two degrees Celsius to flow into the abdominal area. This chemo will be swished in your stomach for two hours to kill the cancer cells. Then they close you up. It is invasive surgery and takes ten to twelve hours to complete, and recovery is six weeks. It is only performed in Toronto, Ontario. He suggested this would be the best, as it has a very good outcome.

This option scared me to death. I was still sore from the first surgery and not fully healed. To cut me open again, check my organs, probe me and then staple me up—this sounded like a nightmare.

Option number two would be taking the chemo drug Fluorouracil (5FU). This chemo drug is to prevent the cancer from spreading and to prolong life. It consists of two chemotherapy drugs, a vitamin and an antibody. It is standard for Stage 4 cancer and given via a PICC line/port-a-cath (hardware is underneath the skin). A chemotherapy cocktail is given over five hours, including blood work. After five hours, you will have a bottle of chemo attached to your port and go home with it. The bottle should empty within forty-eight hours, and a nurse will come and disconnect the bottle.

This chemo will be every two weeks and will continue as long as it is working, with scheduled CAT scans every three months to monitor how well the chemo is doing.

Chemo side effects: nausea, fatigue, sores in the mouth, minimal hair loss. Infections. Bleeding, clotting and changes to your urine.

The oncologist then informs me the information is in the books in my bag the nurse gave me. Also, there is information on a PICC line or port-a-cath, and I will need to decide which one I want.

The doctor says, "I know it is a lot to think about. First, you need time to heal. I will schedule another full body scan within the next couple of weeks, followed by a referral to the doctors in Toronto for the HIPEC surgery. The nurse will call with the date for the CAT scan, and after we have the results, we will go from there." He reassures me by saying if I have any questions, don't hesitate to call.

I was glad Dave was recording this meeting because I am sure when I listen again, I will have questions. The doctor seemed genuinely concerned and compassionate. So much has happened to me in a mere four weeks. I still can't believe this. It is like a bad dream, and I will wake up soon.

It is now just over two weeks since the surgery. I am starting to feel stronger. I am able to walk around the block. Walking is my meditation time. I need to remain positive. I do not want to lose this fight. We went to tell Dad in person what the results were, and I was going to be taking chemo. Still hard to believe. I do not want to die!

June 29, 2018

Dave and Curtis went to work. I feel they are afraid to leave me alone. I spent time looking over the information from the cancer clinic and reading up on colon cancer. I called the nurse at the cancer clinic to see if she knew of any naturopathic doctors I could contact since I was sure I did not want to take chemo. I wanted to seek other options. She could not recommend one. However, she could give me the name of a naturopathic doctor other cancer patients were seeing and asked me to check him out online. The doctor was located in Kitchener, only forty-five minutes away. It was the Friday of the July 1st long weekend. I went online, then sent the doctor an email and explained my situation, mentioning that I did not want to die and asked to book a consultation ASAP. Then, I waited for a response.

I still often wonder if the doctor knew something was not right in Tennessee, and that is why she asked me to make an appointment in six months for another colonoscopy or if my appointment here was sooner, would there have been a better outcome? I need to move beyond wondering and just deal with the situation.

June 30, 2018

I slept well last night and almost on my side. I'm trying to make sure I have lots of rest to heal. My son had some friends over to sit by the pool. It has been above thirty degrees for days, and the humidex feels like forty-four degrees Celsius.

We had a nice visit with my twin sister and her husband. They brought our Dad, and we spent the day by the pool. They stayed for supper. Finally had a bit of real food. My diet has been pretty bland. I had a piece of chicken and a bit of salad. I wanted to see how my stomach was. It seemed okay.

After supper, the guys drove Dad home. My sister, Bonnie, stayed with me to listen to my recorded meeting with the oncologist. As she listened, she started to cry and asked me to turn it off. She felt sick and could not listen anymore. We just can't believe my diagnosis.

I am still struggling with getting comfortable. I am unable to sit for long periods. Standing, walking, and lying down feel best. At night, I struggle with finding a comfortable position. It almost feels like I have to hold my stomach together when I roll over.

The next day, Dave and I went for a walk in the morning. I am walking slower these days, so we walk at the same pace. After the walk, we drove to the market to get some fresh veggies and fruit. Riding in a vehicle is still not fun. I keep a pillow under me for the bumps and on my stomach to protect me from the seatbelt. My stomach is still very tender. We had a very low-key day.

The naturopathic doctor responded to my email with an appointment to see him on July 9. I was surprised as it was Sunday, but it was a perfect way to end the long weekend.

July 9, 2018

Today, we meet the naturopathic doctor. This appointment seemed long. Lots of great information. He is very knowledgeable. He wants to start me on a vitamin C IV as soon as possible. I start next Tuesday since I have a CAT scan today. He answered a lot of our questions. We talked about different options and how the naturopathic methods may benefit my cancer treatment, whichever one I decide on. He did mention the importance of doing both traditional chemo and naturopathic treatments. Dave and I were really happy—finally some hope!

We left his office, and we were off to the hospital for my second CAT scan. Drank the two glasses of barium, then waited an hour. I had to stand and walk because I had done too much sitting, and my stomach was sore and uncomfortable. The scan only lasts about ten minutes. It seems barium liquid does not agree with my stomach, as it causes me to be sick. We went out for something to eat after my appointment, and I had to rush to the bathroom. I will remember this for future scans.

Busy day. Home around 5:00 p.m. I tried to lie down but could not sleep. My stomach was sore and uncomfortable, so I went for a walk. On returning, I sat by the pool and had a glass of wine before going to bed. I slept straight through till 4:00 a.m.

July 10, 2018

When I woke up, my stomach was tender. A nurse from Juravinski Hospital's genetics department called. My sisters and I had undergone genetic testing after my twin sister was diagnosed with aggressive Stage 3 breast cancer. My mom's family had a lot of cancer. We had lost Grandpa and four uncles to various types of cancer. I mentioned to the nurse I had just been diagnosed with Stage 4 colon cancer. She asked me to send her a copy of my colonoscopy report from the clinic in Tennessee. She believes there may be something in our genetics triggering an aggressive type of cancer in our family. When home, I sent her the report and set up an appointment to do more genetic testing next week.

Today, I am receiving my first vitamin C treatment intravenously. I am having this one done in Brantford with the naturopathic doctor who works with the naturopathic doctor in Kitchener. He suggested I go there since it was in my hometown and closer to me. This IV was only vitamin C.

I am glad to have all three doctors working as a team to focus on getting me well. Both naturopathic doctors recommended juicing, so I will purchase a juicer.

This vitamin C drip was only thirty minutes. Since it was my first one, they want to ensure that my body can tolerate it before increasing to 1000 ml. I had a nap when I got home.

July 12, 2018

Woke up after a much better sleep. I had tea, toast, and egg for breakfast and feeling really good today. I went for my morning walk. While I was walking, a cardinal flew right by my head to a small tree. I know it was Mom to let me know she is here with me. My upper back is sore, not sure why. I am now worried the cancer may have spread to my lungs. I will know for certain tomorrow when I get the scan results.

July 13, 2018

Not feeling well today; I think it is nerves. I go to the cancer clinic this afternoon to review my CAT scan results and what treatment plan I will be on. My stomach is sore. Not sure if it is nerves or if I overdid it yesterday. I took some Tylenol and went for a walk. When I got home, there was a message from Hamilton cancer clinic to let me know I had an appointment at 10.00 a.m Monday to have my chemo port put in. I guess this is real. I have cancer and will be starting chemo. Below is the description of the chemo port.

A chemo port is a small, little ball like hardware that sits just underneath your skin. It has a thin silicone tube that attaches to a vein. They put an incision in your neck just above your collar bone. They slide in the tubbing, then the implant ball. It is the size of a large marble and is inserted just below your collar bone. You can see three little prongs like indentations on your skin. The nurses at the cancer clinic like mine because they can line up the port needle and push it into my port accurately, no guesswork. The needle is like a push pin into my port. It has a little plastic tube at the end. The nurse will secure the port needle and the tubing by taping it all to my skin in the area near the port. Once the port is accessed, it will be used to draw blood, hook up chemo, hydration, and on Fridays, my vitamin C IV. The port advantage is that chemotherapy and other medication can be delivered directly into the port rather than a vein, eliminating the need for needles. So for me, it will help save my veins, as you will see going forward. You can swim with your port implant as long as there is no needle in place. The skin over your port doesn't need any special care. You can wash it as you normally would.

At the cancer clinic, the nurse let me know I will have blood work done today (first of many) before I see the oncologist to review my results and find out which chemo treatment I will be taking. I get my blood work done, go to the examing room and wait. My oncologist comes in and starts to review the results from my CAT scan. He tells us the cancer has now spread to my liver and lungs. Again, this was not the news we were expecting. I was no longer a candidate for the HIPEC surgery. Once the cancer has spread to other organs, they will not do the HIPEC surgery. The only option was chemotherapy. The type of chemo is called 5FU and will be given over a five-hour drip. Then I will have a bottle in a fanny pack. It will stay hooked up to my port for the next forty-eight hours. When it is empty, a nurse will come to my home and disconnect it from my port, and I will bring the empty bottle back at my next chemo session.

The oncologist said this type of chemo would not cure my cancer but hopefully slow it down from spreading so quickly. I could not believe what I was hearing. It felt like I was kicked in the stomach. How long do I need to take the chemo? The doctor tells me it is palliative chemo, which means I will take chemo as long as it is working. The next question I asked was about my life expectancy. He replied that with my diagnosis, the average person's life expectancy was six months with no chemo or two to three years with chemo. I looked over at Dave. He was crying. I was trying to keep it together. I could not believe what was I was hearing. I kept thinking to myself, *how can this be?* I had no symptoms. I felt great, and now I could be dead in two to three years? What? This has got to be a bad dream.

The oncologist asked if he should continue. I said, "go on." He suggested I start chemo on July 25. Not the news we were hoping for. He handed me the CAT scan results to read. I was not even sure what I was looking at. Dave and I just listened as he discussed the chemo session, which would be every other week, with a CAT scan every three months to see how the chemo was working.

He asked if we had any questions, but Dave and I were too stunned to have any. He left the room. I felt like I could hardly breathe. In just six short weeks, I have been diagnosed with cancer, had surgery to remove the tumour, found out I am Stage 4 then told it has spread to my liver, lungs, colon, omentum, and lymph nodes. They want to put a chemo port in my chest. When will things finally start to slow down so I can take a breath?

It was a quiet drive home with lots to think about. We cried a lot when we told my son, Curtis. I texted my family to let them know. I kept asking myself, how does this happen when I do not feel sick?

The next day my three sisters and I went to visit Dad. We gave him the news. Dad is a sweetheart who loves his kids with all his heart. Mom died in 2015, so we are everything to him, and he is everything to us. I could not let Dad know how bad it was. I did not want him to worry about me. My dad has enough health issues, so we gave him the short version (not much detail). I am sure my dad knew it was bad. Then we went to see my brother to let him know.

When we got back home, my sisters and I went for a walk, had something to eat, and then they left. I did not do much for the rest of the day. I am still numb thinking about what has happened over these last few days. I still feel very uncomfortable. I have a pain in my left side, in my hip bone. It is a shooting pain. If I put pressure on it, it feels better. Walking this evening was a chore. While I was out on my walk, I stopped over to see my friend, Jerry. I wanted to let him and his wife know the results. Jerry is a very good friend. We are training buddies. We have been cycling, running, and swimming together for years. He is to do an Ironman triathlon in a few weeks. We were supposed to be doing one together. Not sure now. They were both surprised by my results.

July 16, 2018

Slept okay. Still having pain on my left side, so I did not walk today. I am leaving shortly for the Hamilton cancer clinic to have the chemo port put in. I have been fasting, so I am thirsty and hungry. We take my car as it is easier for me. I still need a pillow to sit on to help with the bumps on the road.

At the hospital, I wait in the diagnostics and imaging department. I arrive at 9:30 a.m for my 10:00 a.m appointment since I am unsure where I am going. They were backed up, so I waited until 2:20 p.m before going to the operating theatre. They prep me for day surgery.

When I get to the operating room, they put oxygen on my nose and plastic armrests for my arms so I cannot move them. They do an ultrasound on my neck to see where the vein is and how big it is. They put surgical towels to cover all my hair and my head. They put a cloth over my face. Now I am starting to panic and feel claustrophobic! I keep saying to myself: *Just breathe. You will be fine.* They clean the area, and the nurse begins the drip at the same time. The doctor started freezing my neck. He gets the scalpel to cut my neck and chest, where they will insert the tubing. I can now see the amount of tubing, and I'm thinking to myself, not all of that tubing is going through my neck with me awake! Never going to happen. I ask the doctor, "will you be giving me something to put me out?" His response was "no." He informs me we are just going to freeze the area, and I will be fine. I said, "no, you will need to put me out." The doctor starts to cut, and I jump. Now I am really starting to panic. My face is covered.

I can hardly breathe, and they are trying to put three feet of tubing through a hole in my neck. I say again, "you have to put me out." The next thing I remember was the nurse closing the two incisions in my neck. I was in recovery for two hours. Left at 5:30 p.m. It was a long, stressful day. When I arrived home, I took one of my pain pills and went for a walk.

I then had something to eat and went to bed. I woke up at 1:00 a.m and took another Tylenol. By 5:30 a.m, my neck and chest were tight and sore.

July 17, 2018

I am sore this morning, so no lifting anything with my right arm. Had some green tea, toast, and a pain pill. I went for a walk, and I am still stiff from them putting in my port. The health nurse called with my appointment for a dressing change on my chemo port. She also reviewed what will happen when I have chemo, and they come to disconnect the empty bottle.

Next, off to Kitchener to the naturopathic doctor, who will review my plan now that we know I will be taking chemotherapy. I asked the nurse at the cancer clinic to send him a copy of the CAT scan and the oncologist's recommendations.

My naturopathic doctor is so knowledgeable about the chemo I will be taking. He talked about the chemo bottle I will have with me for two days. He said since my chemo will be Wednesday—with a bottle disconnect Friday—I will start to feel sick on Saturday. The trick to avoid being nauseous is to drink as much water as you can to flush the chemo out of your body. Then, he gave me my schedule of treatments:

Days of the week	Monday	Wed	Friday
Non-chemo Week	1 x 90-min vitamin C/ Mistletoe IV	1 x 90 min vitamin C/ Mistletoe IV	1 x 90-min vitamin C/ Mistletoe IV
Days of the week	Monday	Wed	Friday
Chemo week	1 x 90-min vitamin C/ Mistletoe IV	Two x 60-minute sessions LRHT-Hyperthermia treatments	Two x 60-minute sessions LRHT - Hyperthermia treatments + 90 min vitamin C Mistletoe IV

He recommends fasting, if possible. He informed me my hyperthermia sessions would be on the first day of chemo and on Friday, once the bottle has been removed. I will also receive a vitamin IV during the hyperthermia session. He said, "I know this treatment schedule seems aggressive, but so is your cancer."

Benefits of Fasting during Chemo Treatments:

Cancer patients undergoing chemotherapy may benefit from a fasting-like diet, according to a new study in the 'Medical News Today.' The researchers evaluated the effects of a very low-calorie diet on patients receiving chemotherapy, finding that not only did the special diet improve the effects of chemotherapy but also helped protect the patient's body from cellular damage caused by the treatment.

The cancerous tumor is more likely to shrink, and the patient experiences less cellular damage as a consequence. Researchers found 'significantly' less DNA damage in white blood cells in the fasting diet group.

July 18, 2018

Another restless sleep. Right arm is still sore. I went for a walk before leaving to go to the Hamilton cancer clinic to meet with the nurse about genetic testing.

We talked about my sister Bonnie's Stage 3 breast cancer and my Stage 4 colon cancer and how aggressive they both are. Could we have something in our genes? I did more blood work while I was there and will have the results in three months.

July 20, 2018

Still not sleeping well. I will try moving back to my bedroom from the couch. I can't get comfortable. Bonnie and I went for a walk before she drove me to my naturopathic doctor. This is to be my first vitamin C drip with mistletoe. I pray this helps give me energy and helps my immune system. They start by injecting some mistletoe in my stomach and wait ten minutes to ensure there is no allergic reaction. I did not react, so the mistletoe was added to my IV bag, and my IV was started. Going forward, they will increase the amount of mistletoe they give me. They do this in increments to ensure your body can handle it. I napped on and off during the ninety-minute drip.

The nurse checked my vitals and asked how I was feeling. She was concerned I did not have enough to eat before the treatment. With the vitamin C drip, I did develop a drop in my sugar since I had not eaten enough. It caused me to be lightheaded and dizzy. I asked Bonnie to pick us up a sandwich at Subway. Meanwhile, the nurse gave me apple juice and a nut bar to help with the dizziness. I started to feel better after eating. Bonnie came back with a sandwich. We sat by the car and ate before we started to drive home. I felt much better. The shakes and dizziness went away. Next time, I need to have something more than toast to eat before an IV. On the way home, I started to feel like I finally had some energy. I told Bonnie I felt like I could run a marathon. It felt great to have energy. It was the first time since my surgery I had real energy. Dave was happy but concerned I might be overdoing it.

July 21, 2018

I had a great sleep, and I was still feeling good. Dave and I went to do some shopping. When we came home, I had lunch, then a nap. My port is still tender, so I took a Tylenol.

July 22, 2018

I had a restless sleep. I find it is sore when sleeping on my side. Possibly it could be the port position. I did get up, had a shower, and went to church. I just need not overdo it. Dave had breakfast ready for us when I arrived home from church. I was feeling energetic, so I went for a walk. I will not be napping today. Hopefully, I will be more tired so that I can sleep through the night.

July 23, 2018

Today was another vitamin C IV treatment. I made sure to have something to eat before I left. When I got home, I had some lunch and still lots of energy for a long walk.

July 24, 2018

I am still struggling to find a comfortable sleeping position. I had my coffee and went for my morning walk. When I came home, I had breakfast. The nurse came and changed the bandage on my port.

July 25, 2018.

Today is my first chemo treatment. I arrived at the cancer clinic at 8:45 a.m and weighed in. All cancer patients weigh in for a couple of reasons: one is so when they are getting your chemotherapy treatment ready, they base it on your weight; the other reason is so the oncologist watches for sudden fluctuations in weight to ensure the patient is still doing well. I then filled out the questionnaire on the computer. The questionnaire asks: *how you are feeling, how the last treatment went, are you sleeping, eating* and so on. The nurse has me sit in the chemo room and takes my blood. They send it to be tested. Then I was sent to an examining room. I'm nervous, not knowing what to expect. My oncologist comes into the examining room to review everything. He went over my blood work results, questionnaire, then what will happen today. Before I leave the examining room, he tells me to take my chemo pills. There are eight pills I have to take thirty minutes before chemo. He gives me a prescription for the pills I will take over the next three days. He then hands me a prescription for pills I will need to get for every chemo treatment.

He tells me they verify your blood work is back, and the results are good, before they allow you to take the pills. The nurse explains to me when setting up the chemo IV drip what she is doing and why. It was a long day. I fasted today as recommended by my naturopath. I was dizzy and lightheaded. Five of the eight pills are steroids, so my stomach seemed to be churning in overdrive. I must ask if I can eat something the next time as I need a little food to calm my stomach.

I was exhausted when I came home, so I napped. It was hard to get comfortable with a bottle attached in a fanny pack. I felt a little better after my nap, and I was able to go for a walk. I had been sitting all day, so the walk felt good.

I did not sleep well. I was nauseous, so took some Gravol to help. I am already finding it hard to drink water. I have an early appointment with my naturopath tomorrow. I slept upstairs till 11:30 p.m, then came down and slept on the couch.

July 26, 2018

Woke up at 6:00 a.m after a crappy sleep. I could not wait till morning. Still not feeling well, so I took more anti-nausea pills. Dave drove me to

Kitchener. I took a piece of toast to eat on the way. I was hoping it would help settle my stomach. I noticed I have a new sexy chemo voice. It is so low you can hardly hear me.

Today was my first two-hour hyperthermia session. Again, nervous, not knowing what to expect. It was different; my upper back was hurting by the time the two hours were over. I thought I would sleep, but I didn't. Hyperthermia treatment is different. You lie on a waterbed; then they have this round probe, filled with water and big enough to cover my abdominal area. They position it, and then they lock it in place. It feels like you have a brick on your chest, and you cannot move. This machine sends heated electrodes to the cancer area. It heats up to forty-five degrees Celsius and this is what kills the cancer cells. When the first-hour session is over, they come in and move the probe to the lower area of my stomach. My doctor is focusing on making sure they are getting all of the areas where there is cancer. It is uncomfortable but I know I need this treatment to get rid of my cancer. By the end of the second hour, I have tears in my eyes and my shoulder blades are aching. I can hardly breathe. I hope it will get easier.

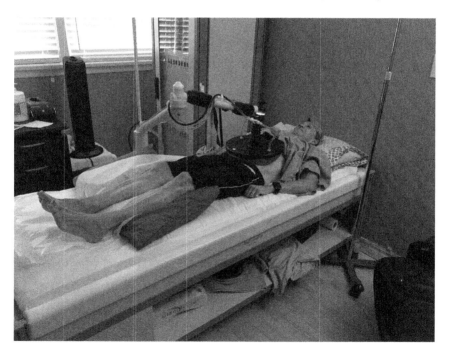

Following the session, I went for my six-week checkup appointment with my surgeon. He thinks I am healing well. He said I look great then said, "see you August thirtieth."

July 27, 2018

It's been a busy week. I went for my walk. I still had my chemo bottle on, but it was now empty. I am glad to have this gone. I still had energy, so I cleaned the house while waiting for the nurse to come and disconnect my chemo bottle from my port. It was nice to be able to vacuum and not have to wait for someone else. The nurse arrived at 11:30 a.m. She removed the bottle and flushed my port. That was pretty slick. The nurse was not long. I had a shower, and this was my first real shower in six weeks. It felt great to have no bandages and nothing hurting!

Today, I am back for my second hyperthermia treatment and vitamin C IV. I got ready and lay down for the two-hour hyperthermia session. For the first hour, I slept off and on. The IV drip was now increased to the normal amount, which was ninety minutes. When the two hours were over, I felt exhausted. I just wanted to go home. On the way home, I was feeling sick and asked Dave to stop for some french fries. Mom always said the "salt and the grease would help me feel better." The fries were so good. I ate them and went for a walk. I was more tired than I thought. It was all I could do to finish the walk. I was dragging my butt. By the time I got home, it was 7:30 p.m.

My sister called to let me know Dad was in the hospital. He had lost his toenail, was on blood thinners, and they were unable to stop the bleeding. While he was at the hospital, they ran some tests. They were concerned his heart rate was only thirty beats per minute and said he would need a pacemaker. Another concern was fluid on his lungs. Dad was sicker than we knew. The doctor scheduled him for surgery to put in a pacemaker on July 31, 2018. Dad is better in the hospital as they will take care of him there. I love that guy. He is a huge humble marshmallow.

July 28, 2018

I slept okay. I was up a few times to take the anti-nausea pill. I walked this morning but ended up with no energy and felt nauseous most of the day. Eating Gravol like candy.

July 29, 2018

I got up and tried to eat something to feel well enough to go to church. I had a shower, but still not feeling well. My brother picked me up, and I got in the truck. When we started to drive to church and were only got a few blocks away, I said, "I cannot do this." He had to turn around; I knew I was going to be sick. Came home, went upstairs, and straight to bed. I slept all morning. I have never felt so awful and had zero energy. I tried hard to go for a walk but could not do it. Things were really rough today.

July 30, 2018

Tried to eat something I could keep down. We had to drive to Kitchener. I was so nauseous. When I got to Kitchener, the nurse checked my vitals and told me I was dehydrated. The nurse started me on a saline IV drip before my vitamin C drip. The hydration made me feel a little better. I was there three hours instead of ninety minutes. On the way home from Kitchener, I was starting to feel like I could eat. We were driving by McDonald's and I asked Dave to stop for a cheeseburger Happy Meal. He looked at me and said, "no way." I looked at him and said yes that is what I want—the fast food I hope will help my stomach. I felt a little better after eating. Still struggling to drink water, though. I can't explain how bad it tastes. It's just not good. When we arrived home, I went up to bed. Still not feeling one-hundred percent. I received an email from my naturopath doctor to call my oncologist to ask him to set up hydration drips on my chemo weeks going forward. He felt this would help me stay hydrated. I am still struggling at night to sleep. Stomach still churning. Slept four hours.

July 31, 2018

Feeling better this morning. I came downstairs had a coffee and a bit of fruit. My voice is starting to come back. I cleaned up the kitchen and went for a long walk. I was a little shaky when I got home, so I had a boiled egg and some dry crackers. Stomach still not right, but I have a bit more energy. Can't drink green tea. Dad had his surgery today to put the pacemaker in.

It's Friday, and I am getting better each day. Managed a long walk this morning. No naps; this will allow me to sleep six to seven hours straight. I went for my vitamin C IV. I was feeling good, so Dave and I drove to Blyth for lunch. I had mushroom ravioli. It was amazing. The drive home seemed very long; it took two hours. I notice I am finding long drives bother my stomach. I moved the seat in the car to try and get more comfortable.

Still having coffee and water for breakfast. No green tea. My appetite has started to increase now that I am feeling better. My stomach must know the fasting is coming up.

August 9, 2018

Chemo treatment number two. There were some adjustments to the amount of chemo to help with my nausea. My blood work showed my white blood cells were low. If they are too low, you will be unable to have chemo. I am at risk of infection when my body's immune system is too weak; it is unable to fight any infection.

I did not feel as dizzy and light-headed this time around. I arrived at the hospital at 8:30 a.m, left the hospital at 1:30 p.m with my fanny pack of chemo, and drove to Kitchener for my two-hour hyperthermia treatment. I am back to Kitchener again on Friday for another two-hour hyperthermia and vitamin C and mistletoe IV. On the Friday's treatments at the naturopath, I was able to access my port. When adding hydration on the weekend, the nurse leaves my port needle in for the hydration IV. With the port needle in the nurse at the naturopath can access my port instead of finding a vein for my vitamin C IV. It is actually pretty slick. Best of all—no needle. With the changes made, this weekend will be the test. I should not be as sick or fatigued.

August 13, 2018

This chemo treatment went much better than the last one, thanks to the recommended changes by my oncologist. He has added a four-hour IV hydration drip on Saturday and Sunday. At my last chemo, on the Friday when I was doing my hyperthermia treatment and vitamin C IV, I could already feel the fatigue setting in. I was sick and felt depressed. I remember lying there and crying through the last hour of treatment. This week was much better. On Friday, they gave me a hydration IV again before the vitamin C and mistletoe. It helped me feel better. On the way home after the treatment, I even asked my sister to stop so we could have dinner. It was wonderful.

I find with chemo that I cannot drink water. The key is to drink as much as you can to flush the chemo out of your body. I normally drink lots of water. Dave has never known anyone to drink so much water. But now, with chemo, I struggle to drink water. I add lemon, oranges, cucumbers. Sunday, I tried carbonated water with lemon. It went down well. I decided that for the next chemo, I will make carbonated water with lemon my drink of choice. I also notice I struggle to drink green tea, which is upsetting because it was my warm drink of choice.

Monday morning, I was nauseous on my way to the naturopath for my vitamin C and mistletoe IV. I took an anti-nausea pill to help make the drive a little better (I have to remember to stay ahead of the meds to keep the nausea under control).

By far, this was a better weekend than the last chemo weekend. I did get the shakes when I was hungry, still nauseous, but I could function. No fatigue.

My training partner buddy, Jerry, did an Ironman at Lake Placid this past weekend. We have trained together for years. He was a big part of my training in 2017 when I did the 200 kilometre cancer ride. Jerry brought me a Lake Placid Ironman coffee cup and gave me his medal. He said once I have completed my cancer Ironman, I can return the medal to him. It was a very touching moment in my journey.

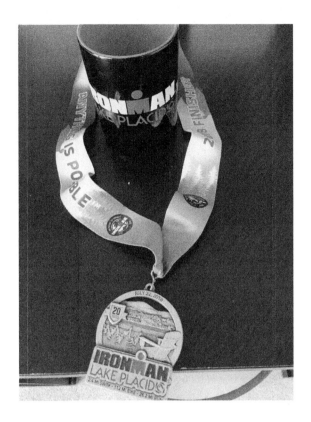

August 19, 2018

After two chemo treatments, I start to get side effects—the sexy voice I now get before leaving the cancer clinic, the sores in my mouth and throat. It hurts to brush my teeth—it actually burns. I have to gargle with baking soda immediately after I eat. I often gargle so I can get rid of the sores before my next chemo treatment. I do not want them to get any worse.

It hurts to eat and drink. I cannot drink anything too cold or too hot. Lukewarm or room temperature is better for me. Dave is getting worried. He sees a lot of my hair on the bathroom floor. I am feeling lucky I have lots of it. If it thins out, that is okay. Less to dry (another side effect to chemo is thinning hair). My sense of smell is in overdrive, so all smells bother me (no more burning candles). Some food makes me sick when I smell it cooking.

My stomach seems to be burning a lot. I find it uncomfortable to sit again. Dave thinks it's because I don't relax. I will call the surgeon on Monday to see why I have the constant burning. I want to ensure I did not tear anything inside.

Other than these few side effects, I feel good. Still walking every day and hanging out in our pool.

August 22, 2018

Chemo treatment number three is delayed a week. I went to the cancer clinic this morning at 8:30 a.m. Checked-in and had my blood work done. Then I went to see the doctor.

My white blood cells were again borderline. If it continues, they may need to reduce my chemo even more, to get these cells back up. I mentioned to the doctor the pain I am having on my right side, just below my ribs. I described it as a burning pain that will not go away. I am still able to function, but I would like to know why I have it. My oncologist noticed on my blood work results that my liver enzyme numbers were four times what they had been two weeks ago. He said that sometimes this happens because of the chemo, so he suggested we delay the chemo treatment until Monday as a precaution. This should help a few things—my white blood cell count should be higher and my liver enzyme count should be lower. If the liver count is still high, he will request an ultrasound to ensure nothing is going on. My liver enzyme count being so high could mean there is an infection. I will go back to the cancer clinic Monday at 8:30 a.m and try again.

I called my naturopath and cancelled the hyperthermia treatments for the week. I decided I will still have a vitamin C IV Friday. He asked I stop all supplements until after Monday's blood work. This will now move my chemo schedule back by one week.

August 24, 2018

Feeling better today. The pain in my stomach is a little more tolerable. I drove myself to Kitchener for my IV drip. Felt good to have some independence. My naturopath changed up the IV, so instead of the vitamin C and mistletoe, I received the following: vitamin C, B-vitamins, zinc, selenium, carnitine, aminosyn, electrolytes, magnesium, and 1200 mg Glutathione.

I was told this combination would help my blood for Monday when I get tested again. If all goes well, I will resume chemo on Monday.

August 27, 2018

Went to the cancer clinic today and had my blood work done. There was no change. The blood was still low and the liver enzymes too high, which means my liver is inflamed. It was not my regular oncologist. He recommended I get an ultrasound on my liver to see why it is inflamed. Ultrasound is scheduled for this Thursday. He suggested I wait another week to get the chemo, review the ultrasound from my liver and my blood work and then decide on the next steps. I am a little worried, hoping that my liver is okay. Now, I wait till next Wednesday.

August 29, 2018

Today, when speaking with my naturopath doctor, he believes the liver being inflamed may have to do with the dosage of chemo. So, I received a gluten drip to help the inflammation. He also started me on a supplement. All of this should help improve the liver enzyme counts and bring them back to normal. Now I pray!!

I cancelled the vitamin C IV but kept the hyperthermia treatments set up for Wednesday and Friday, hoping the ultrasound goes well tomorrow. Also praying my blood work and liver counts are better on Wednesday. Then I will start back on chemo.

September 1, 2018

On Thursday, I went for my ultrasound. The results will be sent to my oncologist. He will review the results on Wednesday with me and Dave.

I have been taking the liver supplements since Wednesday. Today the burning and pain in my right-hand side are gone. I have noticed the bloating in my stomach has reduced. I am feeling really well today. I walked but am still reluctant and do not want to overdo things. I want my blood work and liver results on Wednesday to be great.

September 5, 2018

Chemo treatment. My blood count was better, and so was my liver. I received the okay for chemo. The oncologist reduced the dose, which will help. Thanks to my naturopath doctor, my ultrasound results showed that my liver was inflamed. I am able to get chemo and spent five hours at the cancer clinic.

Right after chemo, off to Kitchener for my hyperthermia. I was there for three hours, which makes for a long chemo day. I am feeling back on track.

September 6, 2018

The past week has been emotional for us all. Trying to stay positive, but it seems we keep getting setbacks. All three of us have done a lot of hugging and crying because of the unknown. Cancer reminds us, "you have no control." We like to be in control of everything in our life—not possible!

I am watching a lot of motivational and spiritual videos. It helps me keep the focus on the big picture. Life is a gift, and the challenges in life are also gifts.

One of the videos sent to me by my sister-in-law, Heather, is called 'Dying To Be Me' by Anita Moorjani. She had terminal end-stage lymphoma. She was in a coma and expected to die on February 2, 2006. The doctors said these were her final hours. She is still alive. I want to be like her.

Here are the lessons we can all learn:

1) Love others but most importantly, love yourself.
2) Live life fearlessly.
3) Be sure to have humour, laughter, and joy in your life.
4) Life is a gift, not a chore. It is only when we lose something that we realize it is a gift.
5) Be yourself. Love who you are. I am working on this.

September 6, 2018

My identical twin, Bonnie, and I have done everything the same most of our life. If something happens to one, it will happen to the other. When I was diagnosed this year with aggressive Stage 4 colon cancer, she said, "Enough with the twin competition. It has to stop." I agree. If it weren't for Bonnie having cancer, I never would have gone in and done all the tests, mammograms, Pap smears, and colonoscopies.

Bonnie has recently completed her Year of Hell. She had been diagnosed with aggressive Stage 3 breast cancer. They found a lump early and had it removed. At first, they expected no chemo or radiation would be needed. That was October 2016. Her surgery was not scheduled until January 18, 2017. She was concerned it may spread, but doctors reassured her that the cancer had been there for seven years. When they finally operated, it had spread into her lymph nodes so now her diagnosis went from Stage 1 to Stage 3 breast cancer. She would need two surgeries, chemo, radiation, and she was very sick during her chemo treatments. She, too, had nothing but bad news at every visit.

She was able to walk me through what my adventure would be. She brought me my chemo starter kit for the house, hazmat requirements, rubber gloves, ginger treats, and bottles of leftover Gravol with ginger. She helped me make decisions about whether to do the chemo port or the PICC. A port was more convenient for my lifestyle, as I wanted to shower and go swimming. She told me to record all of my doctor's appointments. There will be a lot of information, I will be overwhelmed, and I need to listen again a few times to remember. She has been great. I have been able to discuss everything happening, and I have a second opinion. The only thing done differently is I added the naturopathic doctor. Bonnie believes he is the reason I feel so good. It is due to his treatments.

September 6, 2018

At chemo, I asked my oncologist if I could start working out. He explained that being active is important with a diagnosis like mine. I need to be strong and in good shape to help fight the cancer. Anyone who knows me knows that he had just given me the green light to take it up a notch. He did mention doing things in moderation (baby steps and listen to your body). No heavy-duty training for a marathon or a 200 kilometre bike ride. Anything besides walking will be nice once my chemo and hydration are completed. I will put myself on a beginner workout plan. I already have my bike on trainer and have weights, Bosu ball, bands, and roller. I just need to remember to take it slow.

September 8, 2018

Today was our thirty-ninth wedding anniversary, and this was not the way we planned to spend it (we should have been boarding a plane for Puerto Vallarta, Mexico), but we will make up for it next year when it is our fortieth wedding anniversary. We both found it difficult this year to pick out a card. We hugged, cried, and vowed to stay determined to be on the cruise next year.

Today instead, I was off to the naturopath for my 3:45 p.m. appointment—a two-hour hyperthermia treatment and vitamin C IV, with no mistletoe. My naturopath wanted to ensure that the reduction in the chemo is what was needed to get my blood work and liver enzymes back to normal. He stopped all supplements, including my liver supplements, until the next chemo treatment. He is always very cautious.

September 10, 2018

Nausea is back. This past weekend was spent mostly on the couch. I was surprised by the reduction in the chemo mix. I expected to have better hydration drips and hyperthermia treatments. No luck. I felt bad all weekend. I guess the four-week break from my issues with my blood and liver enzymes puts my body back to restart. I did not have much sleep over the weekend. Both days my walks were short and done first thing in the morning before the nurse arrived.

My Monday morning drives after my chemo weekend to my naturopath are always a struggle. I am feeling so nauseous before I go, so I try to eat toast. I get ready, pack my bag with water, Gatorade, ginger ale, apple juice. I need to make sure I have everything. I take my anti-nausea pills, and off we go. It is always a very quiet drive. Once there and after setup for my ninety-minute IV drip, the naturopathic doctor suggested taking ginger supplements three times a day to help with nausea. I am hopeful this will help. When I got home, I headed back upstairs to bed; I had zero energy. I was able to sleep for an hour. I felt better when I woke up and went for a walk to get some fresh air. Things should start to get better now.

September 14, 2018

Consultation and update. I went for my naturopathic treatment, and we met for a status update. He is pleased and optimistic about my progress. My treatment plan is aggressive, and I am doing very well meeting all the appointments even when I am not feeling well. I believe I feel as well as I do because of these treatments. He is very knowledgeable about what I need for supplements, and when I have issues like my liver enzyme levels, he can pinpoint the problem and find a solution. I am grateful!

As he promised, he removed all of the supplements this past week until I got my blood work done on Wednesday. He knew my liver issue was due to the chemo. He also said to give myself credit for my positive attitude and my will for a 'normal' life by keeping so active. He said everything I am doing would only help me fight the cancer. He is very optimistic about my next CAT scan results.

I am very pleased with how well I am feeling right now. I hope my insides are looking as good as my outside because everyone says I do not look like I have cancer (let alone aggressive Stage 4). To me, this is the new look for cancer.

Today, I have slight pain in my stomach. Some friends came for a visit. Got a text from my brother, Alex, to tell me Dad had fallen and was taken by ambulance to the hospital. Alex asked we go to the hospital because Dad was not good. When Dave and I arrived at the hospital, we could not believe what we saw. Dad looked like he had no fight left. We were all standing around the bed as he bobbed back and forth like he was in so much pain he could not get comfortable no matter what we did to help. It was so strange; it was like we were not even there in the room.

Normally, Dad would never let us see him struggle. He was so proud and determined never to show weakness. Whenever Dad was sick, and his kids came to see him, he would cry. Not today. He just looked so uncomfortable, rocking back and forth. Nothing we did seemed to help. I stayed at the hospital until 1.00 a.m. Then my brother-in-law brought me home.

September 15, 2018

During the night, they had taken Dad to Hamilton General Hospital to put in a port for medication. My sisters and brother went to the hospital in the morning. I did not go because of the risk while doing treatments. They FaceTimed me when they were asked to leave the room while putting a port in Dad. They said Dad was not the same Dad. He still did not cry when he saw all of them. They hung up quickly. The nurse had arrived. They assumed it was time to go back and see Dad. Instead, it was because Dad had flatlined, and they were doing CPR. My younger sister (DD) FaceTimed me again to tell me what happened, and they were now in Dad's room. At the time of the call, they were resuscitating him. All I could hear were my sisters screaming to stop because it was too hard on Dad.

Dad passed away at 8:30 a.m. So sad and hard to believe Dad is gone. He will be so happy he is finally with Mom and our two deceased siblings. Michael and Cindy. Later that day, all the family came here to spend time together.

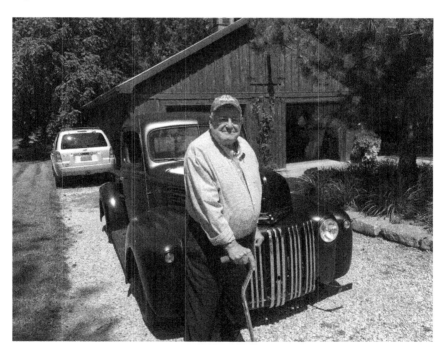

September 16, 2018

Sunday. I went to church with my brother, and it was tough. It was not the same without the big guy. The priest announced Dad had died. My brother, nephew and I took the gifts up to the altar at communion. My family came over again today to my house to be together.

September 17, 2018

I went to Kitchener for my IV treatment. Still, can't believe Dad is gone. When I came home, I went to the florist with my sisters to pick out the flowers for Dad. All bouquets of beautiful red roses. Dad loved his red roses.

September 19, 2018

Woke up, had a coffee, and got ready for chemo. I took a toasted bagel with me to eat with my pills. My blood work was good, and my liver was great. Yeah! Thanks, Dad. Told the nurse about Dad's passing. My oncologist said I did not have to do chemo. I went ahead because I know Dad would have wanted me to have chemo still. I now had another angel to help me from the other side. They reduced my chemo by giving me the a needle with a final push of chemo, instead of my take home bottle. This would be easier at the funeral viewing. They promised I would be finished as quickly as they could. Unfortunately, it took an extra-long time because they accidentally quit one of my chemo bags. This added two hours and delayed my treatments in Kitchener. I was arrived two hours late to the funeral home. When I do hyperthermia, the second hour causes so much stress on the middle of my back. I brought a towel to lie on to help with the pain. It helped a bit, but for the last ten minutes, it was uncomfortable. It takes my breath away when I get up. I continue to plug on!

Hoping with Dad's help, I will continue to get good results and have an excellent CAT scan on October 9.

September 20, 2018

Today is Dad's funeral. Still can't believe he is gone. I went for a walk before leaving for the funeral home. I listened to Dad's song, 'Heaven was

Needing a Hero.' I know heaven has one now. He was our hero!! I took my pills and felt not too bad today. When I got home, I got ready and left for the funeral home. I knew this was the last time we would see Dad. The church was packed. He was a special man, a 'gentle giant.' The church service was beautiful. Dad would have been happy. When the service was over, we all followed his coffin out the door and watched them put his coffin in the hearse. Then, we all watched as it drove away. So sad. All of us walked over to the church hall for the celebration of Dad's life. It was nice to see everyone and talk to them. We got home around 2:00 p.m. It was a long day. I went for a walk to be by myself. When I came home, I lay down. I was exhausted. I felt like everything had finally caught up with me.

September 21, 2018

Hyperthermia treatment today. Today's treatment was long and stressful. Each of the hyperthermia sessions is more painful by the end of the two hours. Today the pain between my shoulder blades was so intense, and by the start of the second hour, I had to ask the nurse to stop. It was so painful I was crying and could not breathe. The nurse had the doctor come in. She was able to do some acupuncture to take away the pain so I could continue and complete the second hour of this treatment. I was thankful!

I have scheduled some acupuncture on Monday as the doctor suggested this would help eliminate the pain for future hyperthermia sessions.

September 22, 2018

Up at 5:30 a.m. Had coffee, apple sauce, took my pills, went for my walk, then waited for the nurse to arrive. She arrived at 9:30 a.m. Felt okay. Had the hydration drip. Felt a little tired and a little nauseous during the day.

September 24, 2018

After a tough week, the four-hour hydration drips worked well. I was not as tired or nauseous this past weekend. The hydration drip seems to go right to my belly and face. They are both so bloated after hydration. I did feel better after and was able to go for a walk. Fortunately!

On Wednesday, when I was at the cancer clinic, they gave me a prescription for a steroid drip that would help with the nausea on Saturday and Sunday. Taking that as a drip along with the anti-nausea pills seemed to work better this weekend. I was still a little nauseous this morning before leaving for Kitchener to see my naturopath to get my vitamin C and mistletoe IV. It feels like morning sickness and lasted until Tuesday. I will know after tomorrow if I am good for a week.

September 25, 2018

People who know me know how important working out is to my daily routine. It has been fourteen weeks since my last real workout. On the Sunday before my surgery, I did a sixty-five-kilometre bike ride. This has been a long time coming. I want to start feeling like I can be normal again. It is tough getting back into it, though. Monday, I started to do weights and stretches (weights only being eight pounds). Woke up this morning with sore legs, but this is a good sore.

It was raining and gloomy today, so I tried spinning on my bike for thirty minutes (I probably cried for fifteen minutes, listening to music that made me think of Dad.) But I did stick it out for the thirty minutes. It feels good to finally workout. I am tired of being sick in the morning, having pains I never had before, being extra cautious picking up or doing anything that could be strenuous.

September 26, 2018

Today I received the IV for vitamin C drip and mistletoe, and afterward, I received acupuncture on my back. The acupuncture was in the mid-back section, which always seems to get knotted up when doing the hyperthermia. The doctors recommended that I have a few more acupuncture sessions to help relieve the pain for future treatments. I was told today no lifting, and my back may be sore over the next couple of days. It was surprising to feel the pop after each needle was injected into my back. Hopefully, I will see good results with my next hyperthermia treatments.

September 28, 2018

Run /walk today. I was feeling good, so instead of my one-hour walk, I did a walk /run. It felt good to get my heart rate up and the heavy breathing while I worked my lungs. It was tough but felt awesome. For all who know me, running is my passion. So, starting to run means I must be getting better. I surprised Dave. He was out walking, and he saw me running.

October 1, 2018

Happy Friday, everyone. October is a big month. My CAT scan is Tuesday.

While at my naturopath doctor, he asked if I would participate in a study**.** He gave me the information on what it was and asked me to think about it - **Bastyr University - Oncology Study for Advanced Stage Cancer Patients.**

I said Yes to participating in 'CUSIOS,' a Canadian /US Integrative oncology study.

This is a five-year study to help assess how well patients do who use integrative oncology services and the long-term effects of advanced integrative oncology care on health and quality of life in cancer patients.

For me, to participate was a no-brainer. I want to do whatever I can to help.

October 3, 2018.

How bad is it when you forget that this is chemo week because you are feeling good?

Today was a good chemo day. My blood work was great, and chemo was a go. My oncologist asked me what my naturopath has me taking now. I told him I just started to take an immune activation liquid, to be taken daily.

He was very happy with everything. He even said I looked amazing.

At the last chemo, he made adjustments and also added a steroid drip which helped. Feeling good today. Left the cancer clinic after 1:00 p.m., then off to see my naturopath. Did the two-hour hyperthermia. This week we started with the lung area for the first hour. I still had the pain in the upper back area. It was really sore by the end of the second hour. The nurse helped me up and had me sit for a bit when I was finished to catch my breath. I think it is lying still for the two hours that bothers me.

Only one hyperthermia this week since I am having my CAT scan on Tuesday. Cannot have hyperthermia close to scan dates because the radioactive waves may disrupt the CAT scan.

October 4, 2018

Not a great sleeping night. I was up every hour. It was a windy, stormy night, with lots of thunder and lightning. Felt sick when I got up but had a coffee and mini-quiches that I made, took my pills, and started to feel a little better. I went for my walk and got caught in the rain again. I have done that a lot this week. Went and got groceries. I grabbed a bowl of soup for lunch. I needed a nap afterward. I was feeling better.

October 5, 2018

I finally had a great sleep. Slept straight through to 4:30 a.m. Felt nauseous when I got up, had something to eat with my pills. Then I started to feel better. I went for my walk. I had a peppermint candy to try and settle my upset tummy. My chemo bottle was not empty, so the nurse will be here at 11:00 a.m today to disconnect my bottle. I was off to Kitchener for the vitamin C IV and hyperthermia.

October 7, 2018

This weekend seems to be going much better. I woke up Saturday at 5:30 a.m and took my anti-nausea pills. I felt well enough to make cabbage rolls for Thanksgiving dinner (my signature dish). Trying to get them done before the nurse arrives to hook up my hydration (success: done and in the oven). Seemed a little more tired Saturday during hydration, so slept lots. It might be the dreary weather making me feel tired.

October 8, 2018

My younger sister hosted Thanksgiving dinner. It was nice to have all of the siblings together. We knew it would be a tough day without Dad.

Getting ready for dinner, I think we all had our 'miss Dad' moments. My sister's moment was when she was making the pies. Dad always peeled the apples and told her what to add to the pie filling so it would taste like Mom's. She had to guess this year. She did a good job because they tasted just right. I am so thankful we have each other, and we are all so close.

October 9, 2018

The day has finally arrived for the CAT scan. I am concerned about my nausea. Would I be able to drink the liquid and keep it down? I grabbed a bottle of water, and we left for the hospital. Checked in to imaging at 7:30 a.m and am not feeling well. The nurse came to the waiting room to see what juice I wanted the liquid mixed into. Apple juice, please (same answer every time). She brought the two beer-size glasses of liquid for me to drink. I sipped slowly until all was gone. One hour later and water for a chaser, I still feel like I could be sick at any moment. Finally, they called me in and inserted the needle for the liquid. The liquid is very warm and travels through your veins, and enhances the organs to show up better on the scan.

My scan in July was not good. It showed that things had spread rapidly. I had five tumours on my liver, and both my lungs had tumours. My omentum had tumours. I am hoping for a reduction in the size and quantity of my tumours. I will not get the results until next Wednesday when I return to the cancer clinic for chemo. The waiting is torturous!

October 12, 2018

First Reiki Session. What is Reiki?
Reiki is a Japanese technique for stress reduction and relaxation that also promotes healing. It is administered by 'laying on hands' and is based on the idea that an unseen 'life force' flows through us and causes us to be alive. If one's life force energy is low, then we are more likely to get sick or feel stress, and if it is high, we are more capable of being happy and healthy.

The word 'reiki' is made of two Japanese words - Rei, which means 'God's Wisdom or the Higher Power,' and Ki which is 'life force energy.

Reiki treats the whole person, including body, emotions, mind, and spirit. It creates many beneficial effects that include relaxation and feelings of peace, security, and wellbeing. Many people have reported miraculous results. I knew for me to get better, I needed to heal mind, body, and soul.

Today, the reiki session was with a very special Reiki Master, Melissa (my niece). I set up this session as another form of healing. I want to fix 'Mind, Body, and Soul.' This will help me to accept my treatments and help get rid of the disease.

I also did Access Bars.

The Access Bars are thirty-two bars of energy that run through and around your head, connecting to different facets of your life. All of the points that you touch when using this modality are called The Bars. They store the electromagnetic component of all the thoughts, ideas, attitudes, decisions, and beliefs you have ever had about anything.

When I was finished, I felt better and lighter. There was a lot of aggression and anger released. The Reiki Master was able to dig deep and bring the problems to the surface so they could be released, and I could start to heal. This was an amazing session.

October 17, 2018

Today we finally received the CAT scan results. My oncologist was very happy with the results. The five tumours on my liver have shrunk, and spots on my omentum and lymph nodes remain stable. My lung tumours are smaller and stable.

The good news is that my other organs and other areas in the body—kidney, pancreas, gall bladder, pelvic, bladder, and thorax—are normal. It is great news that the cancer has not spread. So what I am doing is working. My oncologist was very happy that my blood work was excellent today. I continue to improve. Now off to get my chemo started. I gave a copy of my CAT scan report to my naturopath, who was also very happy with the results.

I will celebrate with wine next week, but for today—a coffee.

October 19, 2018

The two-hour hyperthermia was a struggle. I am finding it harder to get through the two hours. The first hour is tough, but I can do it, then my back starts to hurt. I get restless and am very uncomfortable. My naturopath wants a bone scan just to be sure nothing is wrong.

While I was there, he went over my results and my treatment plan going forward. He said that he realized how costly it was and wondered if I could continue with the same plan until my next scan. My next CAT scan is December 31st at 8:00 a.m. I told him I want to continue the same plan because I hope to clear my liver and lungs. Also hoping my other organs stay clear or stable. I am aware of the cost, but I want it gone! I started back on my supplements.

When I got home on Friday night, Dave and I discussed not doing two hours of hyperthermia because it hurts so much. Will revisit this with my naturopath.

Each chemo is like a fist full of bits and bites. I never know what is in store for me once they disconnect on Friday. This weekend was no different; I seemed okay on Saturday morning, even after my hydration. I went for a walk and slept a little Saturday afternoon. Then, Sunday, I tanked. I woke up not feeling well and was not well Sunday or Monday. I could barely move off the couch. I was so nauseous, and nothing tasted good. I could only drink apple juice, and I had to cancel my IV Monday. I was too sick to be in a car. This was the first time I had cancelled a treatment. Dave thought this one was the worst yet. At 8:00 p.m Monday, I was able to start to drink some water with lemon. Tuesday morning, I woke up feeling better. I will get better each day now until the next chemo. I will be enjoying the next seven days.

October 29, 2018

I discussed my sore back with my naturopath when doing hyperthermia. I told him I was going for a deep massage in my upper back to help with the pain. He said he would continue to do some acupuncture Wednesday before the treatment.

Today while getting the massage, she worked on my left side. She said she could feel the stress. It felt better when I was finished—like the stress had been released. I hope to find it was a success Wednesday, and I will continue to do deep massage before my chemo.

Since I was feeling good Monday, I made my workout a little harder. I ran stairs at the arena close by, along with doing upper body weights and even a long walk. On Tuesday, I increased my walk to six kilometres, then went for a four-kilometre run later in the day. It is nice to feel like I am getting back to what I used to doing, also knowing Wednesday is chemo, so things will go south for the next seven days. I can walk only.

October 30, 2018

Louise Hay had a healing cancer summit podcast that I listened to. It was all types of doctors and patients talking about different types of cancer and how to fight them. It was very interesting. She talked about stress and how it causes cancer, how lifestyle contributes to cancer, what we eat, how we take care of ourselves. She spoke about Reiki and tapping and how beneficial they are for your wellness. I learned tapping in my life coaching training. We did a skill lab on Tapping: EFT, Emotional Freedom Technique or Tapping.

Here is the process. You start at the outer edge of you hand—so the pinky side of the hand—and you'll tap it with two or three fingers and say, "I feel confident, food is peaceful, I am free." You repeat this three times, "I feel confident, food is peaceful, I am free. I feel confident, food is peaceful, I am free." And after those three times, you move to the head. So you go through one side of the body, and then you go through the opposite side. You can do it on one side only, but we did both sides.

The next point you'd go to is the top of your head. Just tap around, "I feel confident, food is peaceful, I am free." Repeat this three times.

Then the eyebrow, that inner part. Start tapping there, "I feel confident, food is peaceful, I am free." Repeat three times.

Then you go to the outer bone. It's kind of like the top of the cheekbone, towards the edge of the eye, kind of where the eyebrow comes down. You start tapping there.

Move down to the bottom inner portion of the eye, tap there.

The next one is right between the nose and the top of the lip. Tap there.

And then the next one is between the chin and the bottom lip. Tap, tap, tap.

Then the clavicle or collar bones, and you're not tapping specifically on the clavicle, but instead, you go down about an inch, and it's the little soft, meaty portion.

Then go down to the bra line essentially, and so for guys, you just go to your sternum, and around and over, but you tap there with four fingers, about four inches below the top of your armpit, about four inches down, you tap there four times. "I feel confident, food is peaceful, I am free."

These last few months have been a learning experience for me. I thought I was doing everything right, but I was not. I hope with what I have learned and the changes I have made, I, too, will be a cancer survivor.

I want to take the experience and what I have learned from this journey to help others, so they never have to experience cancer. Here are some of the changes I have made:

Limit stress; don't sweat the small stuff.

Listen to the body.

Be positive.

Say 'I love you' more often.

Be a hugger.

Live in the moment.

October 31, 2018

I was off to the hospital at 8:30 a.m. I filled out the questionnaire. The nurse struggled to get blood from my port, so we used my arm. Then, they flushed my port so I would be able to use it for chemo. While I was getting chemo, I saw my oncologist. He did not feel I needed a bone scan since I had a CAT scan recently, and everything was good. I mentioned my nausea feels like morning sickness and lasts until noon. He suggested that I take Gravol along with my prescribed anti-nausea pills. I find it hard to swallow when I am not feeling well because I am a gagger. When you feel nauseous, it is even worse. I struggle with even taking my pills before chemo. Today, chemo treatment lasted five hours, and then I was ready to leave with my carry-home bottle. I am on my way to my hyperthermia treatment. It will take another four hours, and then my chemo day is done. Already my voice has started to change to my sexy chemo voice.

Yesterday, I had a thirty-minute deep massage. I am hoping this helps to loosen up my back and eliminate the pain. My Reiki Master sent me a link to 'Healing Angel Message with Archangel Raphael' on YouTube. I will try to listen to it while I have my hyperthermia treatment. I hope that by trying both of these pretreatments, I can get through the two hours. The last fifteen minutes are the toughest.

Well, it worked. Today was the best treatment so far. I will have to try this again for my next treatment. Tonight, I will be back to sleeping on the couch for the next two days while I have my chemo bottle.

November 2, 2018

Today, the nurse arrived at 10:00 a.m to disconnect my empty chemo bottle. I got ready to go to Kitchener; I am hoping it goes as well as Wednesday's treatment. I am already stressing about the discomfort I get with my back.

In the first hour of the treatment, the probe was placed on the lung area and upper chest. I listened to the Archangel Raphael meditation on YouTube, but the last ten minutes of the first hour were already uncomfortable. With only ten minutes left, I asked if we could stop early. The nurse asked me to walk around for a few minutes to see if I could walk off the discomfort. We waited ten minutes so my back would feel better for the second hour of treatment. This time the probe was placed on liver/colon and lower abdomen areas. It was already starting to hurt twenty minutes in. My naturopath had come into the room. He asked me to go with him, and he would try to work on the sore area of my back. He did some acupuncture, added Biofreeze, and massaged the area a bit; then, I went back to the room to complete the balance of the time for the treatment.

I felt better. It lasted about thirty minutes, and again, in the last ten minutes, there was so much discomfort to my back. I will stick it out, though. The doctor found my three favourite songs, the ten minutes were up, and the session was over.

I slowly got up and changed. I was glad the session was finally over for another two weeks. I come back Monday for vitamin C IV. My naturopath suggested more acupuncture and also to try a Chinese method called cupping. It should help with the pain. He suggested that I continue getting the massage before the treatments, hoping this helps relieve discomfort in future treatments. "Praying now, hoping these treatments will help with my discomfort."

November 3, 2018

Another chemo weekend. No two chemo weekends are ever the same. I was able to drink water this time. I added a tablespoon of frozen lemonade. Not sure why, but it works. The water is going down. I was able to get in my seven large glasses of water. When the nurse came Saturday for hydration, I told her that I could drink my water this time, and I did not think I would need hydration. The nurse felt she should do a 500 ml IV and cancel Sunday if I still felt the water was going down well. I was pretty sure I was able to get my water. I felt good Saturday—not too nauseous. I took the anti-nausea pill but only when I got up.

November 4, 2018

Sunday woke up very nauseous, my face very puffy, and feeling bloated this morning. I got up, took my pills, had a coffee and a muffin. Went for a long walk before the nurse came to take out the port connection. I was not doing hydration today. I think I can do it by just drinking my lemonade. The nurse was here a while, then left. I hope I made the right choice. I cleaned up the house, did the washing, had some crackers to try to get rid of my nausea. Not working today. It is a beautiful day just wish I felt better.

It took until 9:00 p.m for me to start to feel okay. Thankfully, I have to be at my naturopath at 10:00 a.m tomorrow for IV, acupuncture, and cupping. I do not want to be nauseous in my car since I am driving on my own.

November 5, 2018

My naturopath was off, so no cupping or acupuncture today; it is rescheduled for next Monday at 8:30 a.m, followed by my IV drip. Next

Tuesday is my appointment for a deep back massage, and Wednesday is chemo and hyperthermia. Next week is another busy and stressful week.

This week has not been bad. My nausea is gone, but I have heartburn that I cannot get rid of. I have not been drinking much water, and my food intake has been bland food—sweet potatoes, boiled eggs, avocado, and protein shakes. I am finding that drinking warm water with lemon allows me to get the fluid I need. With each chemo, I have a new challenge over how it affects me or my taste and smell. I have been doing a lot of walking, stairs at the arena track, and weights at home. I have also been walking with a new buddy this week—Toby, my niece's dog.

November 9, 2018

Reiki session working on alignment.

What is alignment?

Correct body alignment is the optimum alignment where the body is perfectly balanced. Poor posture takes us out of this alignment and is a source of health problems.

By treating yourself to a Reiki therapy session, you receive a full-body alignment with Reiki energy. Reiki energy works with your higher wisdom (inner knowing) to identify how much adjustment is needed within your mental, emotional, and/or physical bodies.

Each session begins with a brief discussion of issues and concerns followed by a Reiki treatment tailored to your needs for balancing the body's energy centres (chakras/meridians) and clearing physical, mental, and emotional energetic patterns that are no longer needed. The session concludes with a sharing of experiences and any intuitive messages and guidance.

My message and guidance were to be more positive about my treatments and welcome them no matter how stressful they seem. I am allowing myself to be thankful for each type of treatment and to feel blessed with every treatment, knowing it is helping to heal my body from the inside out. Having a more positive outlook will allow for more positive results. Reiki helps me realize it is all in your attitude; we need to be more thankful for everything in our lives. So, I will continue to be more thankful for the chemo and the hyperthermia, and with these treatments, I will get better.

So much to learn. I am very grateful for this Reiki session and for teaching me how important it is to be both positive and grateful for everything that happens.

November 12, 2018

Today's treatment consisted of acupuncture, cupping, and vitamin C IV.

My naturopath explained why we were doing this—it will help with the pain in my back on my left side. He is trying to eliminate the pain so my two-hour hyperthermia treatment will not be so stressful. He started with acupuncture on both sides of my neck; then I rolled onto my stomach, and he focused on my left side, where the pain is. He was able to feel some of the pressure release when he inserted the needles. He spent about twenty minutes inserting needles in the sore area.

Then the doctor started to do the cupping. It feels like a suction cup on my skin. It is painful. He adds as much suction as I can tolerate. He did this for ten minutes. He kept going up and down the problem area. After he was finished, he did some more acupuncture. Put on a menthol cream to freeze my back and said he would add this cream to my back Wednesday if it helps me.

He told me no lifting or weights tonight because I would be stiff and sore. I would most likely be bruised in the area he was working on. Since I had scheduled a deep massage for Tuesday, he suggested I reschedule to Thursday. He thought a deep massage after today's treatment would be too much, and I would be really sore on Wednesday. We don't want that. My poor body has been bruised and abused so much in the last four months. I went to the other room so I could get set up for my two-hour IV.

Well, he told me I would be sore tonight, and he was correct. It was very painful driving home. I stopped at my niece's to walk Toby. The walk is what we both needed: me for the pain in my back and Toby just to get out for a walk. It's another treatment I am grateful for and is all part of the healing process.

November 15, 2018

Chemo day went without a hitch. I started my day at home with a prayer to welcome the treatments. They are helping me to heal. My blood work was excellent! My oncologist said I am was good to go for chemo (always what you want to hear). He then gave me a prescription for heartburn. I also cancelled the hydration for Saturday and Sunday this week. So, the lemonade and water had better work. I have faith!

After chemo, I had a couple of hours to kill, so I came home and made supper since I knew we would not be back home until after 8:00 p.m. I did a quick walk and had a coffee. Then off to my naturopath. On the way there, I was feeling a little nauseous; even Dave thought I looked pale. My back was feeling good when I got there, so I was hoping for a good treatment. I made it through the first hour okay. When the hour was up, I got up, stretched, and had a bit of apple juice. The doctor came in to set me up for the second hour. I talked to my sister on the phone; then Dave came in which helped get my mind off my back (thirty minutes have gone). It only started to really hurt in the last fifteen minutes of the two hours. I was not quitting because the probe was working on my liver and I need it to be clear. So, when the doctor came in to see how I was doing, Dave thought I was going to quit, but I said, 'No, I will stick it out." So, I completed my two hours—**perseverance is the key.**

November 15, 2018

Today, I am going for my scheduled deep massage on my back. I am hopeful it will help with tomorrow's hyperthermia treatment.

November 16, 2018

I had a deep massage treatment yesterday, hoping it will help with today's treatment, and I will have no pain. The nurse arrived at 11:00 a.m to disconnect my empty chemo bottle. I got ready to go to Kitchener, and my back was not feeling too bad. When I arrived at the naturopath's, he asked me how Wednesday's treatment went. He was disappointed to hear I was in pain for the last fifteen minutes of the first hour and that the second hour was brutal. He decided that with everything I have been doing, we would only do a one-hour treatment today to give my body a break.

Forty minutes in, I could hardly stand the pain, and the tears started to flow. He came in and said he was going to stop. I said no, I want to continue since we are only doing one hour. What he did was have Curtis put his hand on my left scapula and add pressure to it. It helped relieve the pain for the last twenty minutes. I got through it, but it was slow getting up as usual. He said he would continue with another acupuncture treatment on my week of chemo, along with the cupping. He was also going to give me a needle to freeze the area for the next session to ensure I could get through it. I told Curtis on the way home that my neck was so sore and painful. I think it is stress-related. My niece made up an oil with different ingredients for muscle soreness, put some on my neck on the way home, and by the time I got back to Brantford, the stiffness and burning were gone. *Fantastic!*

I want a week with no appointments, no needles, massages, acupuncture, cupping, IVs, hyperthermia, or chemo. My body needs a break. I have been doing this for four and a half months. My body is tired, and so am I. Sorry, not a good day, and I know my weekend will get worse with my nausea and heartburn.

I am wondering if I am doing too much to heal.

November 19, 2018

It's another interesting weekend. Saturday I was feeling really good. Even did a weight workout at night. This weekend I cancelled hydration because, after the last chemo, I didn't feel I would need it. So far, I am okay with that decision.

Sunday, I woke up around 4:00 a.m feeling very nauseous. I managed to get back to sleep until 9:00 a.m. I got up to shower since my brother Alex was going to bring me communion after church. When I was getting dressed, I noticed a bruise on the left side of my neck. It was the area that had been so sore on Friday night. It looks like the deep massage and cupping were finally coming out. I put the oil on the bruised area that my niece gave me for sore muscles.

I went downstairs and lay on the couch but could barely stay awake. Not able to drink or eat, I just slept. Called to see if the nurse would come and give me the hydration and the nausea drip that the doctor had ordered (which I had cancelled). The nurse never returned my call. I slept the day away. Monday morning, I woke up and felt okay. My stomach was a little woozy but much better than yesterday. I was able to go for a walk today and eat and drink. I will get better each day now until the next treatment. This week is a low-key week. I only have IV on Wednesday and Reiki on Thursday. My body should get some time to recover before the next busy week.

November 22, 2018

Today I had Reiki. It was very healing for me and the perfect treatment to end my calm week. Next week is very busy and hectic. The Reiki Master started with the back area since I have a lot of issues there. Then we switched over and did the front of my body. I feel very rested today, and I have energy. I am in touch with my body much better now. I am more spiritual and have more gratitude and thankfulness for everything happening to help me heal.

November 28, 2018

It will be three days of fasting now while I am on the chemo. It was like every other chemo treatment—arrive at the hospital at 8:30 a.m, weigh in, fill out the questionnaire, get the blood work done. Meet with the doctor to go over how my last chemo went. He tells me my blood work was great. I look great and should keep as active as possible.

Last week I cancelled my hydration, but I will not do that again. Hydration is back on! Then I wait for the nurses to hook up my chemo. I left there shortly after 1:00 p.m, came home, had a coffee, and then off to Kitchener. I received five needles in my back to freeze the area, causing me pain. This method is one used in Germany. The first hour went well. My back did not hurt. In the second hour (my 'witching hour'), I made it through forty-five minutes okay, but the last fifteen minutes were painful, so we ended the treatment early. My naturopath did not think it was worth it for my body to continue with pain. He may decide to put the needles deeper into the muscle, but I won't know until I return on Friday. We left at 5:40 p.m. I had a sore back and a headache. We got home at 6:30 p.m.

I thought I would feel better if I went for a walk, so I walked for forty minutes, feeling much better when I got home. Chemo days are long and exhausting. I have started to sneeze, which means I am getting my sexy chemo voice back.

November 28, 2018

This week has been a busy week with treatments. Routine Monday treatments and acupuncture on my back, tender area on my left side. I can feel the difference in my neck—the left side is tighter than the right. They left the needles in for twenty-five minutes before taking them out. I could feel the stiffness for the rest of the night. No lifting tonight.

November 29, 2018

Today I went to the Brantford Hospice and met with a grief counsellor. Such a beautiful place. Trying to work on my mind, body, and soul. It was a very humbling and spiritual session. The counsellor has asked me to start journaling the tragedies of my childhood and also the happy times. Be truthful. So, that will be easy for me to do. We started to talk about God, spirituality and praying to the saints. Making sure I pray daily, which I am doing, but now it will be with more meaning and spiritual feelings (Mom will be so proud). I showed her I carry Mom's prayer cards—my mom prayed daily. I will now use them. She gave me some holy water to use in my house to remove all bad spirits. It was a very moving session. I think this helped me to realize I need to be a much stronger Catholic, like Mom. I need God's help right now.

December 1, 2018

All these treatments are starting to stress me out. I am never sure what will happen with my back at these treatments. Will I make it through the two hours? Should I reduce the sessions? It is so painful. The drive is always quiet on the way to my treatments. I wonder how much it will hurt this time, how many needles I will get, whether I can make it through the two hours of lying still without crying. Friday is my worst day. It's been a couple of stressful days with my treatments. I know this weekend will be bad; I am overtired. This all takes a toll on my Friday hyperthermia, and

I usually have a meltdown the second hour of treatment where I cry and just want it to be over. I want my life to be normal again.

Today is Friday. It was quite a drive, already not feeling well, nauseous, worried about what will happen when I get to my hyperthermia session. Dave dropped me off. I went in and sat down in the waiting room until they called me in. How is your back? I say okay. Do you want me to freeze it? Yes, I say. I lie down as he put the needles in the sore area. I think it was five needles this week. He set the probe on my liver area for the first hour. My back was okay. It was starting to be uncomfortable, but I was still feeling good after the first hour. Got up, had a drink of water, and a little break before he set the probe on my lung area. He asked how my back was feeling. I said a little tender, so he placed two warmed-up bean bags in the problem area. It helped, so every fifteen minutes, when the bean bags got cold, they would be replaced with a warm one. Yeah! I got through the two hours (but not before telling Dave, "I hate this, and I want it to be over").

The doctor said we would continue to try to figure out why I have so much discomfort on the left side. I just need my CAT scan on December 31 to be good to be done with the hyperthermia treatments.

December 3, 2018

This chemo week, I made sure the nurse came both days on the weekend to give me hydration and a new anti-nausea medication through a drip. This new medication worked well, and within twenty minutes, I felt better, and it eliminated the nauseous feeling for about eight hours.

I changed the amount of hydration down to 500 ml from 1000 ml. I found that after the four-hour drip, I was so bloated—my stomach and face seemed to really swell. Saturday, I was good and still had some life in me. I was able to walk, eat, and went to church. However, I still struggled to drink. Woke up Sunday at 5:00 a.m feeling sick. I could not sleep because I felt so bad. I waited for the nurse to come and give me the anti-nausea meds so that I would start to feel better. I had zero energy; I was not drinking. Tried the lemon water and apple juice. The apple juice went down. I knew I was dehydrated but it is so hard to drink when you are nauseated. It is like there is something lodged in your throat that you cannot swallow.

The nurse arrived at 9:30 a.m, gave me the anti-nausea meds, and then hooked me up for hydration. She noticed a difference right away.

She said my lips were pale, and I looked really tired today. I spent most of Sunday sleeping on the couch. After the nurse came back to disconnect, I decided I would try to go for a walk. Another weekend gone. Monday will be a better day.

Woke up Monday at 5:00 a.m feeling great. I drank a warm glass of water with lemon and finally had a coffee. I told Dave I would not be sitting down today. It is crazy how you can feel so different in just twenty-four hours. I am so glad it is Monday!

December 7, 2018

Another busy week. Started the week not feeling well, but by Wednesday, the nausea was gone, and I am taking pills to control the heartburn I have. This week only IVs—Wednesday and Friday—and a hot stone massage on Thursday. It was nice having no doctor appointments the first two days of the week. I feel I have given my body a pretty good break. Next Wednesday will be the last chemo for this year (I hope longer if my CAT scan is good).

December 13, 2018

Last chemo of the year, and it was stressful as usual. I got to the hospital at 8:20 a.m, was checked in, and weighed. Instead of doing my blood work, I went directly to see the doctor. I waited forty minutes, which delays everything, and my tight window has become even tighter. I will not be finished by 1:00 p.m.

Once I am done, it's off to Kitchener. Once there, my naturopathic doctor and I reviewed a new schedule for IV and hyperthermia treatments (subject to change depending on CAT scan results). More needles in my back to freeze it so my treatments would go well. The first hour and fifteen minutes were pain-free, but then the pain started. The last forty-five minutes were so painful the tears began to flow down my cheeks. They gave me warm bean bags to put on my upper back area for the pain and discomfort. It seemed to help. The pain is on my left scapula, and it is such a sharp pain that it takes my breath away. I lie there on the bed with a probe on my chest and breathe deeply to help me get through until the timer goes off. It was another rough session, but I stuck it out, thinking this is it until January, so suck it up. I completed the two hours, then rested for a bit before I got up, changed and left for home. It was now 5:30 p.m—another long chemo day but the last one this year, yeah! Just one more hyperthermia to get through, then my back gets a three-week break.

December 14, 2018

The day started well. The nurse arrived just after 9:00 a.m to disconnect my chemo bottle.

Off to the arena to run the stairs since it was raining. I had two hours to kill, and I was trying not to stress over my treatment. I told Dave on the way to Kitchener that maybe the naturopath will only want me to do one hour since Wednesday's treatment did not go well (I will be doing my happy dance if he does that).

Well, it happened—this hyperthermia was only one hour. I struggled so much on Wednesday it was best to do only one hour (I was really happy with this decision because I did not think I could do the two hours). Before we started, the doctor did acupuncture needles to help with the soreness and some freezing gel. The nurse set up my IV with mistletoe, and I was ready to start the hyperthermia. Well, I was good until the last fourteen minutes. I had them bring a warm bean bag to put under my scapula to help me get through. This is it for the year, then three weeks off. I was very tired and quiet on the way home. Once home, I had a coffee and some toast. Now I just wait to see how Saturday and Sunday go. Then I have only two IVs for next week. My body will be free of this for three weeks to rest and get stronger.

Hopefully, in the New Year, I will get great news on my CAT scan. I pray the chemo and hyperthermia sessions will be reduced or come to an end.

December 16, 2018

Well, the day has arrived. The nurse disconnected me for the last time this year. I was a little nauseous this weekend, but a good way to end the year. My port has been flushed. I have two more IVs this week, then no more acupuncture, cupping, taking of blood, needles, hyperthermia, or chemo until the week of January 9. I will be a normal person for the next three weeks. I am so excited.

I have a CAT scan on December 31 and will get my results on January 4. I am so looking forward to this break; it will help my body to heal even more.

December 19, 2018

This has been a good week so far. Since I had some free time, I made an appointment with a chiropractor to look at my back (the only thing I had not yet tried). I am focused on trying to heal the left side before January. Tuesday, I went to the chiropractor. He did an assessment and X-rays. Today he made an adjustment, and we reviewed the X-rays. He showed me where my vertebrae were out. It was out in two places—cervical curve and lumbar curve.

The doctor did some strength tests, and my right side was much weaker. This is what is causing the stress (pain on the left side). I go again tomorrow for another adjustment and again on December 24. Hopefully, this will be the final piece to help me heal. After the chiropractor today, I went directly for my IV, then home. Tomorrow it is the chiropractor and then off for a Reiki session.

December 22, 2018

Reiki Session. This session was my last, so it was a little different. Melissa (Reiki Master) talked about affirmations and how they reflect on self-growth. My homework was to create my personal affirmation (I need to start with 'I Am.' She asked me to dig deep within myself.) Melissa started with a prayer since prayer was very important to me at this time.

Melissa started by working on balancing all of the chakras (soul balancing), which will help to complete all the other body balancing that I have been doing. As she worked through all of the chakras, she went through affirmations. This Reiki session was perfect. With all I have been doing, I feel that I really have started to heal mind, body, and soul.

December 22, 2018

Friday was my last IV for this year; I go back on January 2. These IVs have helped me so much. I have more energy.

December 23, 2018

My week has been amazing. I think my body is already starting to feel better. I have two more weeks. Awesome!

December 30, 2018

2018 has come to an end. I had an amazing Christmas; I have been enjoying the break. I feel NORMAL. I have been able to work out each day, which some people may think is overdoing it, but this is normal for me. Tomorrow is my CAT scan. I am a little nervous but feeling very optimistic. My son knows how much I love angels, and for Christmas, he gave me two sets of angel cards—one is Angel Therapy, and the other is Guardian Angel tarot cards. So today, I pulled one from each box. Feeling more optimistic after I read these cards. All the hard work I did is paying off. I will find out for sure on January 4.

PART 2

Continued Treatments 2019

January 4, 2019

I met with my oncologist at the cancer clinic today to review my CAT scan results. The tumours on my lungs are unchanged, and my lungs are otherwise clear. Great news! The tumours on my liver reduced in size—one went from 7.6 mm to 5.4 mm; the others went from 7 mm down to 2 mm, 7 mm down to 3.5 mm, and 6.6 mm down to 4 mm. All my other organs are normal.

I would have liked the cancer to be gone, and I will need another three months of chemo, hyperthermia, and vitamin C. I had my blood work done today and back to chemo on Wednesday.

January 9, 2019

Chemo day. My blood work was done, so chemo went pretty quick today.

Home by 12:30 p.m, then off for hyperthermia. I am only doing one hour, with hopes it will help the pain in my back. Also, getting back adjustments at the chiropractor. Forty minutes into the treatment and my back was starting to hurt. It was hard for me to breathe, but I was able to stick it out. Feeling good so far. No nausea yet (touch wood). I do have my sexy chemo voice and sneezing like I have allergies. Tomorrow back to the chiropractor. Friday disconnect of chemo, hyperthermia, and vitamin C and mistletoe IV.

January 13, 2019

Chemo weekend. On Friday, after my disconnect, my older sister came with me to my treatments. To add excitement to the drive, I got a flat tire. No problem, my older sister was there. She took control, and we made the appointment on time. Hyperthermia is still a struggle. I only seem to be able to stand it for forty-five minutes. I had no freezing or acupuncture this week. I thought my appointments with the chiropractor would improve my back strength, but they didn't. The nurse gave me a warm bean bag to help me get through the treatment. I did not help; I was still in a lot of pain. I will discuss what we can do for the pain on Tuesday with my naturopath when we have my follow-up meeting. The nurse was here Saturday and Sunday to give me hydration and an anti-nausea drip. I had zero energy this weekend. It was all I could do to walk Saturday for thirty minutes. I came home, had some supper, slept in the chair till 10:00 p.m, then went to bed. Sunday, I got up and had some warm water and lemon. Then, off for a short walk before the nurse arrived. The nurse hooked up my hydration and gave me the anti-nausea drip. I slept in the chair for three hours. I am disconnected now and have zero energy. Hopefully, tomorrow will be better. I am not recuperating as quickly after my break.

January 15, 2019

My naturopath was very happy with the CAT scan results. He said the results were awesome, and I should be very happy. I said I hoped they would have been clear. I guess it was a little unrealistic to think Stage 4 aggressive cancer would be gone in six months. So yes, I am a little disappointed. I did thank him. Because of his plan, my tumours are shrinking, and my lungs are clear. My naturopath said he helped, but it was "my all or nothing attitude." He does not want me to lose my drive and determination to beat this. He said the fact I am eating well, working out, and trying to remain positive is a huge factor in why I am doing so well.

He mentioned, "Do not look too far ahead. Be happy with each milestone." He said my next CAT scan still may not be clear. His concern is I will get depressed. He wants me to maintain my great drive and positive attitude. Getting these results is excellent for my diagnosis. He said he had had many patients fighting for eight years before remission. Then he reminded me again to not look at six months down the road but one week or one month at a time.

We then reviewed what we need to do to help me get through hyperthermia treatments going forward. We went over supplements to take to help with nausea and lack of energy during chemo treatments.

This was a reality check for me. I have been treating it like training for a race. However, in this race, I have come to understand I have no control. I need to stay strong and be positive every single day.

January 24, 2019

Well, this chemo day was stressful. Long day at the cancer clinic. As usual, I'm always watching the clock to ensure my treatment is completed, so I can leave there to go home for a coffee before my hyperthermia treatment.

On the way to my treatment, I can already feel the stress in my back. I put an oil on my wrists for stress relief. Curtis gave me a pocket pharmacy of oils to keep in my purse. There are oils for headaches, the immune system, digestion, stress, and pain relief. I used the 'digestion' on my throat when I got home to help with the nausea. When I got to my hyperthermia session, my naturopath inserted ten needles in my back to numb it. It should help me get through the hour (glad I am not doing two hours). He also added a small water pillow for me to lie on. I was able to get through the session. Still, I had pain the last few minutes, but it was tolerable.

I am sneezing again and still able to drink my water. My sexy chemo voice is back. I never sleep well when I have the bottle attached. I have the bottle until Friday when the nurse comes to disconnect it. When lying on the couch to sleep, I can smell the chemo, and it bothers me. I try to make sure I have covers over the chemo port access, but I still smell it.

January 26, 2019

I was at my chiropractor in Cambridge, Ontario. My right side was weak, and he was working on making it stronger. I have attended five sessions now. It has been painful, and my right side seems stronger; however, the pain on my left scapula will not disappear.

January 26, 2019

The nurse arrived at about 9:30 a.m to disconnect the chemo bottle. I went for a walk, then off to Kitchener. The drive was not bad. It was snowing, so we left a little early. Again, I am stressed knowing it will hurt, and the drive to Kitchener is quiet. I start feeling my back tense up, and my stomach is upset—not sure if it is the chemo or stress. I got in to see the nurse for the IV hook-up and the needles to freeze my back. They tell me hyperthermia treatments are thirty to forty minutes behind schedule—not what I wanted to hear. I am stressed and upset, knowing it will be after 4:00 p.m; by the time I am finished.

I asked her to skip the needles today. I am just not feeling it. Please just load on the freezing gel and hope it gets me through the hour. Dave dropped me off and did not bring his phone, so I know when he gets here, he will think I am almost complete, and I have not even started.

It is almost 3:00 p.m. I have the IV hooked up, my back is frozen, and I am cold. The hyperthermia room is almost ready for me. I get in, lie down, the nurse sets the probe, puts on the music, and we are ready. I started forty-five minutes late. The nurse leaves, and I am by myself. I start crying, thinking how I hate this. I want it all to go away. I am so over all the needles and the driving and the stressing. I just want to be normal. I start to pray, asking God to please help me get rid of this disease. When Dave arrives, I tell him to check the time on the machine. I had fifty minutes left. "Behind today. Sorry for the delay," I said. Dave responded, saying we do not have to be anywhere, so relax. With those words, I fell asleep. I woke up with less than twenty minutes left on the machine. There was not much pain— a little discomfort, but I was okay. I was finished now for two weeks. Quickly, I got up, dressed and said my goodbyes, and went out to meet Dave, who was waiting in the truck.

I was feeling a little better to be "done." Talked a little on the way home and then made us pasta for supper. I cleaned up, sat down in my chair to watch the rest of the news, and fell asleep. I was exhausted.

January 27, 2019

I am not feeling bad. The nausea drip I have been doing before hydration is helping quite a bit. Even though I wake up not feeling well, by 9:00 a.m, after my five-minute drip, I start feeling better. My hydration is only three hours now, reducing by an hour, so I am not as bloated and puffy. Still struggle to drink water. I always have a large glass of water and lemon. I did find out this morning that this anti-nausea drip makes you tired. That explains why yesterday I felt tired after I was disconnected. I ended up going for my walk but felt exhausted when I got home.

After a stressful Friday, this weekend has not been bad. Sleeping a lot, getting lots of rest. The nurse will be back at noon to disconnect the IV and remove the needle that accesses my port. Then I will be FREE. Looks like a beautiful winter morning. I can't wait to walk later today.

February 2, 2019

My naturopath thought using some medical cannabis might help me when taking chemo. It will help with nausea, pain in my back, sleep, and stress. I sleep on the couch Wednesday and Thursday nights when I have my chemo bottle attached. I can smell the chemo from my bottle when I sleep, which makes me nauseous. I went on to the cannabis website, set up the appointment, answered the questions online. I had an online interview with the nurse about cannabis and why I need it. I was approved. She talked about which type of cannabis would help me. I went on their website and purchased my prescription of cannabis in a spray form. The nurse set up a follow-up appointment in a month to see how things were going and if I had any questions.

Still a little nervous, but talking to other cancer patients, many use the drops and have had success with them. Hopefully, it will help me with the anxiety and stress on Wednesday and Friday with the chemo and hyperthermia treatments.

February 6, 2019

Chemo today: did not drive on to Kitchener. I rescheduled the appointment to Thursday. I will be doing back-to-back hyperthermia. My cannabis has arrived. I did use the nausea spray. I was a little scared, but I was not feeling well and thought, this is great, try it at home. The type I am using is sprayed under the tongue. It did not taste great. They recommend you take it with a piece of cheese. The spray works in about fifteen minutes and lasts three to four hours. The other spray I purchased is for pain and stress. I will try it later tonight. I am keeping track to see how I feel. This process will help me figure out the correct amount to take. Cannabis is another learning curve for me.

February 7, 2019

Last night was a restful night until 2:00 a.m. I could not get back to sleep, so I opened up the cupboard to try my new spray to help me get back to sleep. It did help; I slept through to 5:40 a.m when Curtis woke me. It helped eliminate all the tossing and turning on the couch. I took the spray again just before we left for my hyperthermia treatment. It seemed to make me more mellow. Still a quiet drive to Kitchener, but no stress in my back yet. I asked the nurse to use the freezing gel on my back still. I lay down, and they started the machine. I fell asleep right away, made it thirty-five minutes into the treatment. I woke; I was not feeling too bad. I just lay there and said my prayers and waited for the session to be over!

On the way home, feeling rested, we stopped for groceries. Still feeling good, I cleaned the house. However, this is only Wednesday; the test will be Friday, my bad day. The time when the chemo bottle is disconnected, the nausea kicks in, and so does the stress.

February 8, 2019

Today was the test with the cannabis. As I said, Fridays are my worst day for treatments (I cry, more stress, anxiety, and pain.) This Friday, I used my new cannabis spray. I took it about twenty minutes before the treatment. I was not as stressed on the drive there, and my back did not hurt as much in anticipation of the treatment.

When I got there, the nurse put the freezing cream on my back. I felt more relaxed. We went into the room, hooked up my vitamin C and mistletoe IV, set the probe to the centre of my stomach to cover the liver, lungs, colon, and omentum. I said my prayers to welcome the treatment and fell asleep. I woke up because my mouth was dry, and I needed a drink. I only had twenty-four minutes left. Dave came into the room. This was a good treatment; the cannabis helped. What a difference this treatment was. A few weeks ago, I told Dave I didn't think I could continue. This week I feel better and will continue till the cancer is gone. When I got home, I felt good enough to go for my one-hour walk in windy weather—just feeling good!

Tomorrow will be the test with the nausea spray. I am not getting the nausea drip this weekend. So far today, I am able to drink my lemon water, and I am not feeling sick yet. Usually, about now, I am starting to go downhill. But again, no two treatments seem to be the same.

February 10, 2019

Chemo weekend. This weekend, I tried the cannabis spray to help with the nausea. It helped a bit. I took it in the morning when I got up and again at night before going to bed. During the day, I took my nausea pills. I was a little nervous using the spray because I drive to church Saturday night since I am unable to go Sunday morning. I can feel the difference in about fifteen to twenty minutes. It only lasts three to four hours, and then I start to feel crappy again. What I noticed this weekend, though, is I have no energy after hydration. I sleep a lot—could my body be taking in the treatments? I finally got off the couch at 4:00 p.m and did my hour-long walk. It felt good to be outside. I'm feeling a little weak since I struggle to drink. Back home, I had a small Gatorade, hoping the worst is over and I will start feeling better.

February 11, 2019

Great week. This is my non-chemo week. Each day I feel better. I did a lot of walking, had a few slips on the ice. It felt good to walk with my special four-legged buddy, Toby.

I did some workouts and a spin class from YouTube downstairs on my bike (wow, I thought I would die, and it was only the twenty-eight-minute class). So, I need some work on that, more cardio on my good days. Will not be running with all the ice outside.

February 20, 2019

Chemo day. Finally, a day with no stress. My Uncle Art and Aunt Sharon were also at the cancer clinic today. Art was getting his first immune therapy treatment. I finished today and was out before 12:30 p.m.

I took both cannabis sprays—one for nausea and one for stress—before I left for Kitchener. When I arrived at my naturopath's, I got ready for the treatment. Then they put the cream on my back to freeze it. Set up the hyperthermia; no music today. I slept through the treatment. Yes! Right through the hour. OMG!! It worked.

Dave said that he wouldn't come into the room when the nurse said I was sleeping as he did not want to bother me. Today seemed so quick and painless. We were home by 4:30 p.m. Awesome day. Thanks to my guardian angels for allowing me to accept this treatment to help fight the disease.

Friday's hyperthermia treatment. The nurse arrived at 11:00 a.m to disconnect the empty chemo bottle, which starts my cycle of going downhill. Before I left, I took the cannabis for nausea since I was beginning not to feel well. When I was almost there, I took the spray for pain. I was not feeling well on the drive there. Beautiful day for a drive, and we got there early. I thought, great, maybe I will get in early. I was told I looked tired. I said it was the drugs. I was hoping for a repeat of Wednesday. We went into the room, turned off the music. I said my prayers and fell asleep for thirty minutes. I woke up and needed a drink. My back was starting to get sore. It continued to get more uncomfortable through the next thirty minutes. Not as painful as the previous session—just uncomfortable.

Still not feeling great on the way home. When I got home, I went for a walk, still feeling tired. It was so beautiful out I could not stay home. Walked my six kilometres, had a large glass of lemonade, and sat on the couch. Still feeling tired. I know it will be an early night. My back is sore as I am writing this. Again, I will need to try something a bit different in two weeks. I am still learning how to find the correct dose. It will come. Hoping the hydration goes well this weekend.

February 23, 2019

Hydration day one. I woke up not feeling well. The coffee did not go down so well, so I tried tea with honey and lemon. Not good, either. Tried the cannabis this morning before I went for a walk at seven o'clock. I did not feel much better. The nurse arrived at 8:30 a.m to hook up my IV and back to disconnect at 12:30 p.m. After the nurse left, I went over to my niece's and walked her dog, Toby. I thought the fresh air would make me feel better. Came home, sat down, and watched Netflix. I had some chicken in hopes that the meat would help me feel better. Got ready for church with my sister. I went to church still not feeling well. Stopped on the way home for some regular Gravol. When home, I took a pill and went to bed. Hope for a better day tomorrow.

February 24, 2019

Hydration on Sunday is my worst day. I took Gravol, anti-nausea pills, and cannabis, but I could not shake the nausea. The nurse arrived Sunday at 8:30 a.m and said, "You are not feeling well. I can see it in your eyes and your colour." She said my eyes were glossy, and my face was really pale. The nurse said it was a big change from Friday. She said I looked great Friday. Again, spent the day on the couch sleeping on and off. No walks Sunday. Even as I write, I am still nauseous. I cancelled my appointment with my naturopath for tomorrow.

I cannot go in a car right now. I was sick brushing my teeth. The drink of choice for this chemo is Gatorade. I took Gravol this morning to settle the stomach. My last two chemo weekends were tough. Both weeks I did not take the anti-nausea drip. I will ask my oncologist to start them again. I am still trying to find the right dose of cannabis to relieve the nausea.

This was the toughest chemo weekend in a while. I was still sick Monday. It has been a while since I was down and out for three days. I woke up today feeling not bad; nausea was gone, and coffee tasted good. I have this burning in my throat I can't get rid of, though. The good thing is I am now able to drink ice water, and it is soothing my throat. My voice is getting a little hoarse, so I am unsure how this new side will be. Good news is I was able to walk today. I have been house-bound for the last two days, so it was awesome to be outside. Toby was as excited to see me as I was to see him.

February 27, 2019

Today I went to my naturopath for vitamin C and mistletoe IV. I told him about the burning in my throat. He told me it was a side effect from the chemo, and it would probably continue to worsen with each chemo. He told me to start taking zinc and also recommended a throat tea with marshmallow root and also slippery elm lozenges. I bought everything he suggested and took the zinc pills on the way home. He said not to drink anything too hot because it would irritate my throat more. I am drinking water with ice. I also mentioned to him that I seem to be getting sicker after each chemo. Not bouncing back as quickly. He said that it was my immune system getting weaker (not what I wanted to hear). I consider myself to be strong. I guess after seven months of chemo; your immune system starts to break down. He also mentioned that my oncologist would probably suggest a break from chemo after my next CAT scan to build up my immune system.

March 4, 2019

I went for my vitamin C drip IV. On the way home, I stopped off and took Toby for a long walk. I think we both needed it. I stopped at the arena and did stairs, knowing I will be feeling crappy later this week. I am a little worried about Wednesday—chemo day.

March 6, 2019

Chemo went as planned. Good blood work. Chemo is done, and I was out by 1:00 p.m. Off to my hyperthermia treatment. I took the cannabis before I got to my appointment. It helped with the nausea. The nurse put the freeze gel on my back. With the freeze gel and cannabis, I was able to sleep through the hyperthermia. A good session. I am still a little tired but not feeling too bad.

At the cancer clinic, I spoke to my oncologist today, and he ordered the nausea drip and hydration for this weekend. Bad news, though—he is taking medical leave starting Monday, so I will be getting a new oncologist.

My niece, Nicole, asked me to watch a show on Netflix—*Heal*—it is worth watching. The movie is about holistic healing and conventional medicine. After watching it, I am more confident that what I am doing is right. It is healing the mind, body, and soul. There was a cancer patient on there with Stage 4 cancer who is now cancer-free. I want to be like her!

March 8, 2019

Good day. I got up and had my chemo meds. Felt a little upset in the stomach, so I took the nausea spray. The nurse was here early to disconnect the chemo. She left, and then I went for a five-kilometre walk, came home, and showered. Then off to Kitchener. I took both sprays on the way. Once there I went to the room to change, waited to get my IV hooked up and the freezing on my back, and then off to the hyperthermia room. I lay down with the probe on my stomach. We were ready to go. I said my prayers and slept through fifty minutes. I woke up because my mouth was dry. My IV and hyperthermia ended at the same time. This was the best Friday treatment. Maybe I have figured out how much to take (with both sprays, I did one and a half sprays).

By the time I arrived home, though, I was tired. I had a coffee and rested. No walk with my buddy Toby today. I am hoping for a good weekend of hydration and not so much nausea.

March 11, 2019

Saturday was good. Did not feel bad. Did my walk after the nurse left and went to church, still feeling pretty good! Around 8:00 p.m, I started to feel sick. Sunday, I was sick when I got up, and I rested for most of the day. No energy. My neighbour brought over supper, so I had a little bit of food, still not feeling well. Went to bed around 8:30 p.m. Woke up at midnight and was sick to my stomach. Still not feeling well this morning—big headache and can't eat anything. Once I get rid of this headache, I will go for a walk to feel better.

March 19, 2019

I went early to get my blood work done today, as requested by my doctor. The nurse called to tell me my blood was low, and they would have to re-do my blood tomorrow. If it is still low, there would be no chemo this week. I received an IV with more nutrients which will help my blood work. It is so great to have two doctors to work with.

March 20, 2019

I went to the cancer clinic at 8:00 a.m as they requested so I could be ready to re-do my blood work. They told me yesterday it was borderline at 1.4. Today my blood was even lower at 1.1— it needs to be 1.5-7.5. I have been maintaining anywhere from 2.5-2.7. So, I was sent home. No chemo this week (the doctor is concerned if I get sick, I will have no immunity to fight back). I will go back on Wednesday, April 3. My CAT scan is next Tuesday, March 26. I am a little concerned about what the results will be. You know you can look and feel good, but it is no guarantee of what is going on inside.

I cancelled the hyperthermia sessions for today and Friday. My naturopath suggested I take a Deep Immune formula and to get some astragalus and take this together, so it will help build my immune system.

March 26, 2019

My CAT scan today. I am hoping the results are good. I will get my results next Wednesday before chemo. Today I pulled my angel card. It was Archangel Raphael—The Healing Angel (perfect).

I have been seeing red cardinals a lot this past week (Mom and Dad), so tonight, when I walked, I asked Mom and Dad if they were with me during the scan to fly by and let me know. Then two red cardinals flew by! Then, I saw this affirmation on Pinterest today before leaving for the hospital :

March 26, 2019

'God is turning your situation around right now. You are not damaged goods. God is still going to use you and shape you into the woman he has predestined you to be.

AMEN'

So, the signs are showing me it should be a positive!

April 3, 2019

Chemo day and the results from my CAT scan. The news was excellent. My liver is unchanged, and my lungs, colon, omentum, and lymph nodes are also unchanged. Dave and I went expecting the worst, and we were so happy we cried. The doctor said three more months doing what I am doing and maybe have a chemo break for a month or two. My oncologist was very happy with the results, as was my naturopath. I will celebrate with dinner next week. Awesome news! I will be one hundred and fifty percent better over the next three months. I am kicking cancer to the curb!

Dave left, and I went to the chemo suite to start my chemo. Chemo days are always stressful. I do my blood work on Tuesday, thinking this may speed up the process. But no, I still spend most of my time watching the clock and the window where the chemo comes out. When at the cancer clinic, I often am asked about naturopathic treatments. Most patients are so impressed with my results and how I look. I seem more energetic and positive. I often get asked, "who am I here with?" The patients do not think I am there for treatments. When I let them know I have aggressive Stage 4 colon cancer that has spread through my abdomen, they are very surprised.

Today, one of the nurses told me I have changed over the last eight months. I am more accepting of the chemo treatments (thanks to my Reiki Master, who explained how important it is to welcome treatments).

While I was receiving my chemo treatment, one of the nurses asked me to spend some time with a new patient who had just been diagnosed. This person was very special to that nurse; it was her mom. I went over my cancer diagnosis and what my treatments were with my naturopath. The cancer patient had just been diagnosed with Stage 4 colon cancer. She and her husband were very excited and want to call the naturopath and set up an appointment. I handed them one of his business cards and said how amazing he has been; I am doing well because of his treatments.

When I arrived at my naturopath's, I handed a copy of my blood work and a copy of my CAT scan results. I asked her to have the doctor check out the CAT scan. I went and changed and got ready for the hyperthermia treatment. The nurse came into the room to freeze my back. I told her the great news, and she gave me a big hug and was so happy. She said she would get my doctor so I could tell him personally. My doctor came into the room, and I shared the great news. He was happy with my results and said I should have a glass of wine tonight to celebrate. My treatment was a blur. Adrenaline had kicked in. We were all so happy. When I got home, I went for my six-kilometre walk, and I spoke with Bonnie to share the good news about my results. I told her my doctor said I could have a glass of wine to celebrate the good news. She cautioned me not to drink until I feel better and reminded me I was on an adrenaline high with a possible crash and burn soon. She was right; I was asleep by 8:30 p.m.

April 5, 2019

The nurse was here this morning at 10:00 a.m to disconnect my chemo. I made a nice tuna sandwich before heading to Kitchener for treatment. Fridays, we usually use my port which makes it easy on me as I don't need to endure any more needles.

However, it seems my naturopath received a notice that naturopathic clinics can no longer use port access for treatments. So I had my IV started in my arm. She said my veins were thin today—the start of dehydration. The nurse put the freezing gel on my back, and it was off to the room for my hyperthermia treatment. Once I lay down, she set the probe on my chest, then started the machine. I slept almost straight through the hour. My doctor came in to see me when I had ten minutes left. We are booked for a consultation on Monday to review the CAT scan and make any changes he thinks will help. I am always more tired on Friday. I slept off and on during the drive home. When I got home, I felt I should go for a walk. I did my six-kilometre walk, then had a nap on the couch.

Hoping tomorrow is not going to be a bad day. Saturdays are pretty good until about 8:00 p.m; then I am sick until Tuesday. We'll see what happens this weekend. It will be warm out, so maybe the sunshine will help me stay motivated and keep me moving. Today is Curtis's birthday (my rock).

Cancer clinic called with a date of my next CAT scan—June 19 at 7:40 a.m. Great time for me.

Chemo weekend. I got up and went for my walk before the nurse came to hook up the hydration. I was not feeling well, so I took some Gravol. I also did the cannabis spray. I am drinking a fruit juice which seems to be going down. I am still feeling sick, so I do not want anything to eat. I slept off and on most of Saturday, then finally went to bed at 5:00 p.m. I slept through till 1:00 a.m then got up for more Gravol. Still sick and weak with zero energy. The nurse came Sunday to give me hydration treatment. I still had little energy; I think it is due to no food. I slept off and on Sunday. Around 2:00 p.m, I decided to go for a walk. It felt good to get outside, but still feeling a little lightheaded. When home from my walk, I had a sandwich. That made me feel better, and then I napped. Monday morning, I got up at 3:00 a.m. I was going to be sick. Still not feeling well, I took some Gravol and rested on the couch. When I woke up at 8:30 a.m, I was feeling a little better. I made a coffee and had some applesauce. More Gravol.

April 8, 2019

I asked my older sister Helen to drive me to my treatment. I cannot drive. My naturopath will be going over the CAT scan results today.

He was very happy with the results and made no suggestions for changes at this time. Confirmed the next CAT scan is June 19. If my next scan is still clear, then I will be able to take a break from chemo. A break from chemo! Hurray (even though it would be a temporary break). I will continue to have CAT scans every three months. He plans to continue hyperthermia treatments, IV, and supplements. I told my doctor I would do whatever it takes to get a break from chemo. My next milestone is my CAT scan on June 19.

My family and I are so happy with this latest CAT scan result. I have to thank my entire medical and naturopathic team, the cancer clinic team, and everyone who has given me the love and support since my diagnosis last June.

April 10, 2019

When I was walking this morning, I was thinking about the meeting with my naturopath when we talked about my scan and what I still needed to do. I said that this cancer has been like training for a marathon or any other race that I have trained for. You figure out the race you want to enter (cancer would not have been my choice), then you put together a training plan. You follow the plan and train as hard as you can until race day. You want to ensure you are strong when you finally cross the finish line. This is exactly what I am doing—training for the toughest race ever. But I will cross the finish line strong.

April 12, 2019

Dave took me out tonight for dinner to celebrate my excellent CAT scan results. We went to Juniper Dining in Paris (Ontario). It was a quaint restaurant. The food was very good. After dinner, we walked around Paris. It was so nice out tonight. We are so happy with the results. I just need it to continue. I love the celebration but still cannot let my guard down. I know it is not close to being over yet.

April 12, 2019

IV therapy today. While waiting for the ninety-minute IV drip to complete, I sit in a room with seven recliners. I see the same people. Sometimes I bring my iPad and read, sometimes I nap. But most days, there are a bunch of chatty cancer patients. Today was one of those days. I was with four other cancer patients, who I see often. This is like our therapy session. We talk about our scans, celebrate milestones, talk about chemo treatments, our doctors, new treatments etc. I am the only one doing chemo in this group today. Most of the patients at my naturopath are Stage 4.

Today's group: two of the ladies today had breast cancer and have been clear of cancer for three years and continue with IVs as maintenance. Another lady had breast cancer; she never did chemo. Now she has a large tumour on her spine. She had been in the hospital this past week and was released on Thursday. She had been getting daily radiation to shrink the tumour before they could operate. This new tumour was causing her a great deal of pain. It made it hard for her to walk. She struggles to do stairs. I was glad to see her today, but what a difference in the three weeks since I last saw her. I felt so bad when I saw her. Unfortunately, she died shortly afterward.

The other lady was seventy-four and had uterine cancer. Her hair had regrown, and she was still trying to get used to the new hair. She was telling us about this test she had done called a CEA test. This blood test tells you how many active cancer cells you have in your body. Her levels were as high as 438, and my naturopath helped treat her successfully, decreasing to eight. She informed me it had been escalating over the past three months, so she is scared that she will have to start chemo again. She is an amazing lady. I am going to ask about this test. I would consider this a benefit. One thing for sure is that we are all in agreement; we are doing well because of the treatments we are receiving from our amazing naturopathic doctor.

April 17, 2019

Chemo day. This morning before I left, I went outside to see if Mom was out there. I could feel her around me. There was a beautiful red cardinal sitting in the neighbour's tree. I said, "Good morning, Mom," and went up for my shower, then got ready to leave. Mom was with me, so I knew this was going to be a good day.

Today was the quickest chemo ever; I was finished by 11:30 a.m. I did my blood work yesterday, which I think helped. I was able to come home and have a coffee before travelling to Kitchener. At the cancer clinic, I spoke to a new cancer patient. She informed me she had made an appointment with my naturopath. I assured her she would be really happy. She shared she had a bad couple of weeks. No chemo last week because she had a fever, and today no chemo because her blood count was low.

I arrived at my naturopath's, lay on the bed, and said my prayers to welcome today's treatments. I remind myself these treatments will allow my body to be strong and healthy and help fight this cancer disease. I fell into a nice sleep and slept for most of the hour. As I reflect, these sessions are becoming noticeably easier. I still struggle with nausea, sneezing, sexy chemo voice, and fatigue. Again, I am not able to drink water, so I am drinking apple juice. Once I finished my juice, I went for my walk. It is a gorgeous day. Tomorrow is back for a treatment because of the holiday.

April 22, 2019

I had hydration for three days instead of two. I thought three days of hydration would help me with the nausea, even though I still took the cannabis and some anti-nausea pills. The effects were short-lived, only lasting till Sunday. I tried orange Gatorade instead of my regular apple juice, as I was not eating. I hope it will help me with the shakes and lightheadedness.

I slept most of this weekend, experienced zero energy. I truly was sick the entire weekend. I woke up this morning. I did not feel too bad, so came downstairs for a nice cup of coffee. I could not drink it. I grabbed my coat, a peppermint candy and went for my walk. When I came back, I felt a little better, although my stomach is still gurgling and upset. The daily walks help a lot when I am not feeling well. The peppermint candy really helps to settle my stomach, as does the fresh air. Thankfully, I notice I am feeling a little better.

April 23, 2019

Today has been an amazing day. Had a great sleep. Coffee tastes good. I started back on my prescribed supplements. While I was drinking my coffee, I was sending daily affirmations to my sisters and some friends. While sending them, I came across a saved affirmation, which I've posted below (April 28). When you read it, you will know why I pray every day. I was so surprised; I showed it to Dave and Curtis, then I sent it to my sisters, knowing they would know where it came from. There are miracles!!! God is listening to my prayers. March 26 was my last CAT scan.

When I walk, I always say my prayers! When I am finished, I talk to Mom, Dad, and my deceased siblings, Michael and Cindy. I am closest to them when I am outside. It is my time to meditate and focus on healing, gratitude, and positivity.

April 28, 2019

I spent the weekend with my twin sister. I went to her hairdresser in Toronto for a consultation to see if I could get my hair coloured. This hairdresser specializes in colouring chemo hair. She did my sister's hair after she was finished chemo. It has taken nine months to get it to the colour it is today. She told me I still have chemo in my hair. She would not colour it now as there is a high risk I could lose my hair. I am not willing to take the risk, and neither was she. She suggested we wait until I am finished chemo, which will hopefully be in June. She did say it would be a gradual colour change and would probably take nine months to get to a colour like my sister's. I made an appointment for July 13. I am feeling excited.

Orangetheory Fitness. While I was at my twin sister's, she took me to her new gym —the name is Orangetheory. This gym does interval training.

The two of us went to a class on Friday and today. We worked on the treadmill, rowing machine, then did floor exercises. There is a board to show if you are in your "zone." This helps to ensure that you are meeting your target heart rate zones. It was awesome. I loved it. I felt so normal. I was working as hard as everyone else. It was great that no one but the trainer knew I was fighting cancer.

"Life is too short to wake up with regrets, so love the people who treat you right, love the ones who don't just because you can, believe everything happens for a reason, and if you get a second chance, grab it with both hands. Kiss slowly, forgive quickly. God never said it would be easy. He just promised it would be worth it."

May 2, 2019

I did my blood work on Tuesday again, and I'm waiting to see if my blood work will be good today. On Wednesday, I fill in the questionnaire, weigh in, and do a urine sample so that they can test my liver. I waited to see my oncologist. He told me my blood work was borderline as always, and my liver enzymes were excellent. Chemo started early without any glitches. I was finished by 12:30 p.m—only four hours this week. I had time to come home for a coffee before leaving for the hyperthermia treatment. After the freezing gel was applied to my back, I lay down, said my prayers, and went off to sleep. If my mouth did not get so dry, I would be able to sleep right through the hour. Still feeling good, I met my older sister at the arena on my way home to walk on the track since it was raining out.

May 4, 2019

The nurse came early Friday to disconnect my chemo bottle; then, I was off to Kitchener for hyperthermia and vitamin C IV. I felt pretty bad after the disconnect and took the last of my chemo pills. I was quiet on the drive. I took the cannabis on the way there. When we arrived for my treatment, I asked the nurse if I could use my port. My veins are not as easily accessible as they used to be, and they now have to use the veins in my hands. I am bruised quite badly. Unfortunately, she was still not able to use the port.

My doctor is not allowing for port access. There was a complaint sent out to all naturopathic clinics. They are now no longer able to access patients' ports. Darn! Port access makes it really easy for me since my port is active already. No prodding my hands or arms trying to find a good vein. The intravenous needle was inserted successfully into my vein in my forearm. It is a smaller vein so we need to slow down the IV. This IV will be longer than the hyperthermia. She then froze my back. I lay down and she positioned the probe on my chest and breast area to ensure she has targeted my full stomach/liver/lung area. The machine starts; I say my prayers and fall asleep. I slept most of the hour and then waited for the IV to finish. Still a quiet drive on the way home. When home, I went upstairs to bed for two hours. Woke up, had something to eat and then walked at 7:30 p.m. I was feeling better. I am finding I am more tired with this chemo. I have not been as nauseous, but it is still early.

May 4, 2019

Woke at 5:45 a.m as the birds were so loud. I had a coffee, still not feeling bad. Dave said I looked good today. Not nauseous yet. I did my six-kilometre walk, had a shower, and waited for the nurse. She had my hydration hooked up by 9:00 a.m, which was great. I will be finished by noon. I hope to stay feeling good. I plan on taking Toby for a nice walk this afternoon once my hydration is complete.

May 5, 2019

This Sunday was like the others (worst day of the weekend). No walk this morning before the nurse got here. Feeling sick. I was sick just brushing my teeth. I took my anti-nausea pills, had the nurse give me the anti-nausea drip before hooking up my hydration. Feeling really tired, so I rested on the couch after she left. Toby stayed with me on the couch. I slept until my brother came over to give me communion (around 10:30 a.m). After he left, I went back to the couch and slept until noon when the nurse came back to disconnect the hydration. I was starting to feel a little better, and I was able to have a coffee. Yeah! I took Toby for a walk. When I got back from my walk, I was feeling tired, so it was back to the couch. I spent this weekend on the couch feeling really tired and weak.

Thank goodness tomorrow is Monday. This weekend is over, and I know Monday will be a better day.

May 9, 2019

Off to my naturopath for IVs. The treatments are getting harder on me. The nurse is finding it harder to find a vein. Lately, she has been putting the IVs in my hands. She switches each time to a different hand. Since last July, I have received between two to three vitamin C and mistletoe IV treatment sessions per week. This does not include the needles for drawing blood or the chemical they give me for CAT scans. Lots of needles are starting to take a toll on my veins. A vein develops scar tissue if used often, so an alternate vein must be found. I told Dave when I got home Wednesday, "I have to be clear at my next CAT scan so that I can take July off from both chemo and my IVs." My veins need a break, too.

May 12, 2019

Happy Mother's Day to all. I hope you have a wonderful day. My son spoiled me again and gave me the book *Complete Wellness*, which is very interesting. This book has a lot of great information. I found information on supplements to take to help my immune system and blood count. Some of them I am already taking, but there were a couple I wasn't. I have added them to my shake (I am always worried about my blood work being low, so we will see what happens). Thanks, Curtis. Love you.

I did it. I joined Orangetheory gym. I have to work this into my schedule so that I can go four times this month. Today's interval training was awesome. It was based on endurance. I do not have much endurance right now, so this will help me get stronger. It is great to feel normal again. It was such a great workout. Just changing it up and getting that sweat on again is incredible. A great Mother's Day. When I got home, Curtis made me oatmeal pancakes. Feeling so blessed today.

May 17, 2019

I did my blood work on Tuesday before going to my treatment for vitamin C IV. I am always anxious when I go in for my blood work, always waiting for the call from the cancer clinic to say my blood work is 'not' good. I did not get a call this week. My blood work was actually better than the last one. I did a couple of changes this past week, adding more supplements to help to improve my immune system and blood cells. I added to my daily intake some astragalus, ashwagandha, turmeric, along with the Deep Immune. I also take vitamin D and zinc. I think the changes helped my blood work. I will continue this going forward. With these supplements and the vitamin C combo that I get from my naturopath (IV includes vitamin C, potassium, magnesium, mistletoe, cancer-killing supplement, and calcium), I have a lot going in this body to ensure that I stay healthy and continue to be active and feel good.

The only downfall to the vitamin C IV is my veins have been taking a beating, but it's all for a good cause.

Chemo day went without a hitch. Blood work was good, so I was able to take my chemo pills right away, then wait for the chemo to be administered. I have three drips and a needle to prevent cramps and vomiting. Between each chemo drip, they run a ten-minute flush through my body before setting up the next bag. When it is all finished, I get my chemo bottle that I wear for the next two days. It took four hours today— best time. I came home, had a coffee, and off for hyperthermia treatment. The hour went by pretty well; I was fortunate and slept most of the time. My usual quiet ride to and from Kitchener. Dave is getting used to no talking. I came home, had a nap, and at 6:00 p.m went for a nice walk.

May 18, 2019

Up at 6:00 a.m. Had my coffee, did my crossword, and then off for my walk at 7:00 a.m. I wanted to have my walk and be showered before the nurse arrived. I also wanted to have some breakfast. I had a poached egg with avocado on half an English muffin. The nurse came at 10:30 a.m to disconnect the empty chemo bottle. My hyperthermia treatment was at noon today. My younger sister drove me today. I am still able to get some water down, so not feeling bad yet. The coffee is not good today. I reminded myself the coffee would be shitty until Tuesday. I look forward to Wednesday—'best cup of coffee day.' The hyperthermia treatment went well. The freezing of my back helps me a lot, as does the cannabis I also take before my treatment. Maybe I am just getting used to the drill. I was tired when I got home, so I had a nap. Then at 4:00 p.m, I got up and had a coffee to try and get moving. Habit—even if the coffee is crappy. I made supper and afterward went for another walk. Need to take in all these nice days. Hopefully, I will have an okay by the weekend and not be so nauseated. Every day I wake up, it is a whole new ball game. I really am getting used to this drill. That is scary.

May 19, 2019

This Sunday was like the rest. Not feeling good when I got up. No coffee. I only did a short walk, feeling quite nauseous. The nurse arrived just before 9:00 a.m—same old routine. I was still feeling tired and sick, so after the nurse left, I rested on the couch. I did not wake up until noon when she came back to unhook the hydration. I felt much better. I actually told the nurse I was going to have a coffee because I felt so good. She said I looked much better than this morning. After my coffee, Curtis and I went to get some groceries. When I returned home, I went for a walk and even washed my car. Feeling better. I guess I needed the sleep.

May 23, 2019

It was one year ago today that I was in my doctor's office and got the news that no one wants to hear, "you have cancer." I do not remember much after that. I remember sitting in my car saying, "what the fuck just happened?". Then calling Dave on the way home, still not believing what had happened. The weeks following were a blur. I was someone who was never sick and now going for surgery. Every time we went to the doctors, it was more bad news. A lot has happened this past year. I always think back to what Mom would say, "God only gives you what he thinks you can handle."

It has been a challenging year, and I have learned a lot about myself. I am so grateful to my parents, who taught me to be strong and never give up. Love you, Mom and Dad, and I miss you so much.

May 27, 2019

Today I finally got out on my bike, thanks to my friend who checked over my bike to make sure that it was ready to go. It has been a year since I have been on my bike. My last ride was sixty-five kilometres the day before my surgery last June. I was a little nervous this morning at the start, but once I got going, it felt great. I am trying to get some kilometres in so I can ride the last twenty kilometres of the two-hundred kilometre 'Conquer Cancer' ride in June with my niece and my neighbour. The ride is over two days on the weekend of June 8—one hundred kilometres on the Saturday and one hundred on the Sunday. They are both riding. I am so proud of them. I will be there at the finish to support them. I did the ride in 2017 in honour of my twin sister, who had breast cancer. This year, my niece and neighbour are doing it for us both.

June 1, 2019

My chemo this week has not been bad. My blood work was good on Tuesday, so no delays with the chemo. I keep worrying about the blood work. I have not mastered my worry, and I'm always waiting for a phone call. The hyperthermia went well on Wednesday, but Friday's was uncomfortable. My back was sore, so I tried to move but could not do it. It seemed like a long hour for my vitamin C drip. The drip actually took an hour and a half. I felt increased fatigue and slept on and off from Kitchener.

June 2, 2019

At chemo on Wednesday, they showed me a new port needle. It was much smaller needle than the port needle I had been using. I tried the smaller one out. It seemed to be fine. My chemo went through at the same time. This weekend the nurse came to give me hydration treatment, and the port needle did not seem to work as well. She thought maybe it wasn't long enough. After you use the port, they put two syringes of saline to flush the port, and then they push through Heparin (to prevent blood clots). The next time they come, they pull back the Heparin until they see a little blood come back in the syringe. Then they flush with saline (which is a saltwater solution). Saturday and Sunday, they pulled back, and nothing came out. I stood up. I put my arms up and nothing. Then she tried for a few more minutes—a little more saline, then pulled back, and it finally worked. Some blood came back, thank heavens. The nurse was happy, so then she set up the hydration IV. After she left, I had a nap on the couch and woke up three hours later to see I had only got about 200 ml instead of the 500 ml required. We think it is the new needle.

Not sure if it was the position of the needle in the port when I was sleeping. I will let the nurses know at the cancer clinic when I am back on June 12.

June 3, 2019

I slept most of the day. I did go for a walk after the nurse left. Then I slept until 5:30 a.m Monday. Feeling better today, not so weak. I had a Gatorade on the way to my 8:00 a.m appointment for my yearly mammogram. When I got home, I went for my walk. Feeling much better. I just need a good coffee. LOL.

June 8, 2019

Today is the start of the two hundred-kilometre ride for cancer. My niece and neighbour are doing the ride. I was supposed to do it, but there is always next year. They are both en route now! This ride has raised over twenty million dollars for cancer. This is the twelfth year, and more than 5,000 riders are participating. It starts at the BMO Field in Toronto and ends day one at McMaster University in Hamilton. Tomorrow they will start at McMaster and finish at Niagara Falls.

I want to thank both for participating in this ride. Great job, ladies!

I rode this morning. Only thirty-three kilometres, but it was great to get out on the bike again. I went riding with my cycling friend, Jerry. I got a new automatic gear shifter installed on my bike, thanks to Jerry!! What a difference. It is so smooth shifting gears and makes hill climbing much easier. I am very excited to be back to cycling.

June 9, 2019

Today was day two for the cancer bike ride. We went to Niagara to be at the finish line for my niece and neighbour. The ladies did an amazing job. It was a beautiful weekend for the bike ride. While we were waiting there, Dave and I signed up for next year. **"I will ride as a CANCER SURVIVOR."**

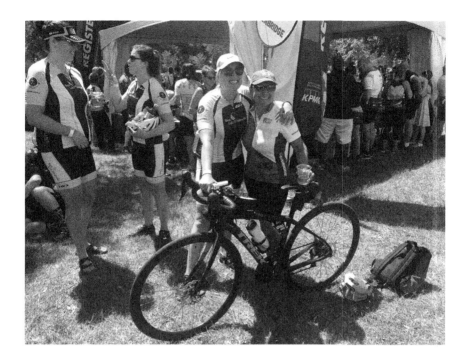

June 12, 2019

Tuesday morning. I went to the cancer clinic and had my blood work done. I told the nurses the new smaller port needle did not work so well at my last chemo. The nurse struggled to pull the blood back, and also, my hydration did not work on Sunday. They put the old type of needle in my port this week. Took my blood, and I was off. If there is no phone call, I am good for chemo Wednesday. I left, came home, and did a thirty-four-kilometre bike ride. This will be my last workout for a week. Still feeling really good.

June 12, 2019

Chemo day again. Stressful. I am always watching the clock because I have to go to Kitchener. I do not like to be LATE! Reviewing my blood work, I noticed my liver enzymes had doubled this week. I asked my doctor, and he mentioned it could be the chemo. The type of chemo I have goes through the liver. I wanted to be sure that it was not due to my increased exercising. He assured me it was not (I did not want Dave to take away my bike or workout shoes). I am good and in the clear. I did, however, mention it to my naturopath. He suggested I start taking my liver enzyme pills Monday with the rest of my daily supplements.

For my hyperthermia treatment, I asked the nurse not to freeze my back. I am going to try it without the gel. I slept most of the hour. It still hurts when I try and get up after my treatment. Then, when I get in the car, I always feel tired on the way home.

The good news is that I will not be taking chemo again until July 24. Dave and I agreed that I need a break. I spoke with both doctors today, and they agreed and were happy with my decision.

Next Wednesday is my CAT scan, and talking with my doctor, who also goes on holiday starting next Thursday, we will go over my results in July when he returns. I wanted the results sooner but am still hopeful the news will be great.

Next Thursday, I will go for another mammogram exam. For this one, they insert dye as they do with the CAT scan to be sure that there is nothing there. Lots of results are coming to me in July.

June 14, 2019

Great nurses. The nurse was here by 9:30 a.m to remove the empty chemo bottle; then, I travelled to Kitchener for hyperthermia. The nurses are all amazing at the cancer clinic (VON Canada) and my naturopath's clinic. They all support me and my tight schedule to ensure I make the next appointment on time. On the weekend, they know I am hooked up to a pole for IV for three hours, so they try to come as early as possible. I say, "Kudos to all the nurses and the hard work they do." Without them, my treatments would not be the same. I want them to know how much I appreciate the amazing job they do.

June 17, 2019

It was one year ago yesterday that I came home from the hospital after my surgery. I remember it was Father's Day, and I could not wait to leave the hospital and get home. It has been a wild and crazy year. When I sit and think about how much has changed, I still can't believe it.

This past chemo weekend was like the others; I was not nauseous but very tired. On Sunday, I went for a walk after the nurse left, came home, took some anti-nausea pills, and went straight to bed. I slept till 5:30 a.m. Sleeping it off is the best medicine. It took me a while to learn not to fight it. I am so glad this was my last chemo for the next five weeks. This break will help me get better each day. This week is a busy week—hyperthermia on Tuesday, CAT scan on Wednesday, mammogram with dye on Thursday, and hyperthermia again on Friday. Next week, things start to slow down, and it will be my time to do what I want.

I am looking forward to getting up each morning and not checking the calendar to see where I am going or what time I have to be there. It will be five weeks of Orangetheory and cycling. I can't wait!

June 21, 2019

I have now completed the last appointment from this busy week. Today will be my last vitamin C IV for three weeks. I am on holiday! The only appointments are Orangetheory, an oil change for my car, and a hair appointment. It is going to be an amazing three weeks. I will start back at hyperthermia the third week of July and back to chemo on July 24. This will be a change to what I have been doing over the last year. I am so looking forward to getting up, having my coffee, and not having to rush off to a doctor's appointment. I am so excited!

June 22, 2019

Today was for Mom and Dad. Our family got together to put Mom and Dad in their final resting place. They are just a stone's throw away from Michael and Cindy's gravesite. It is nice to know that Mom and Dad are finally together. They have been waiting for this since Dad died last September.

Love you, Mom and Dad. Miss you every day.

June 25, 2019

The mammogram is normal. Last Thursday, I had a mammogram with a dye injection so they could have a clearer view. The doctor's office called to let me know it was normal, and I will be scheduled yearly for my mammograms. Great news. I was nervous!!

I went to the hospital today for my blood work to test my liver enzymes (ALT and AST). My liver enzymes were double after my last chemo. Last Monday, I started to take the liver enzyme pills I received from my naturopath. It helped the last time my liver went 'south.' I just wanted to ensure they were helping this time. I await my results with my fingers crossed!

ALT is an enzyme found in the liver that helps convert proteins into energy for the liver cells. When the liver is damaged, ALT is released into the bloodstream and levels increase. Aspartate transaminase (AST) is an enzyme that helps metabolize amino acids.

June 28, 2019

On Thursday, I met with my naturopath to go over my future plan. He said I need to continue with all of the supplements I am taking, stay active, and eat a healthy diet. While I am on this break, I will continue intermittent fasting (I do this when I take chemo). He also commented on all the hard work I have done this past year. Never missing an appointment, even if I was sick. Always giving more than a one hundred percent willingness to try anything to fight this cancer, no matter what. Even when it's painful, I still kept going. This is why it is paying off. No one would even know I had cancer. He said I should be proud of myself. He said this was a well-deserved break, and he was happy for me. I need to enjoy myself. My body needs it. I asked about working out every day. He gave me the green light to do what feels good. He tells me to listen to my body, and most of all, have no regrets. As a cancer patient, you never know what is in store for you. So I will seize the moment and focus on enjoying my workouts and taking time for spiritual moments.

When I start back in mid-July, I can drop down to one vitamin C IV per week. YEAH! We won't make any changes to the hyperthermia until after I receive the CAT scan results. I was happy with the appointment. I hope my call from my oncologist next week is just as positive.

June 28, 2019

Week one of freedom. This week went by quickly. I worked out at Orangetheory every day. It was awesome to workout like I used to. We finished this week with the Mount Everest workout on the treadmill. Now for the long weekend, we are holding our yearly Canada Day pool party on Saturday, and then I plan on cycling Sunday and Monday.

It was a great week of no needles, no chemo, no stress. I know the few weeks will go by fast. I am trying to enjoy every minute of my time being normal. I hope everyone has a great Canada Day weekend. The weather is going to be amazing. Enjoy it!

Sunday, I cycled with my cycling friend Jerry again. It was great to get back to riding. Today Jerry was riding to Dover; I opted out of the ride and did a smaller one. I rode to Dundas, Ontario, and back—only fifty-five kilometres. Now I can enjoy the rest of Canada Day by the pool.

July 2, 2019

Results from my CAT scan are in, and my liver is clear.

My lungs are still unchanged. I am told it was an excellent CAT scan. I should be happy. I continue to take chemo. I will start back on July 8. Dave and I spent a couple of days cycling in the United States. We were in Niagara Falls (US side), drove to the Finger Lakes, and stayed at Glenora Wine Cellars and Inn. It was nice to get away and do some cycling together. We have not done that for a few years. The weather was great, the cycling and scenery were awesome.

July 23, 2019

I was a little worried when doing my blood work today because I have a head cold. It started Sunday night with a sore throat. By Monday, I still had a sore throat and runny nose. After supper, I was all stuffed up and could not stop sneezing. Yikes! I cannot have chemo when I have a cold or am sick. I was scared to take anything last night. This morning my head was so full, my stomach felt awful, I had an achy body and felt really tired (all symptoms of a cold). I slept until 7:00 a.m, then had a shower, and went and had my blood work done. On the way home from the cancer clinic,

I stopped at Metro to get some Tylenol Cold. I took one of the pills and slept until 10:30 a.m. Woke up feeling better, had a drink of water then finally went for my walk. No call yet from the cancer clinic, so I think I am good to go for tomorrow. I just need to rest today.

July 24, 2019

Back to chemo today. One year tomorrow since I started the chemo journey. The nurse gave me my blood work results; it was fantastic today. It must be all of the Orangetheory workouts (four times a week), the cycling, and the rest time. It has paid off.

Today, I sat beside my uncle Art at chemo. It was quick today—out before noon. I experienced some hiccups. The nurses had to take my blood pressure five times today because the readings were too high. They also struggled to get blood from my port.

My blood pressure might have been high because of my talk with my oncologist. When he came into the room, he said, 'your scan was excellent; you look great." I still had some questions about my CAT scan and also about my chemo treatment. I needed to understand what the actual CAT scan meant in terms of cancer-free—my ultimate goal! There were five tumours on my lungs, and they have not changed. There are still tumours on my liver. However, there is no change which is a good thing. To me, when I got the news 'clear,' I thought that meant everywhere. But I am not clear everywhere. The next question was, "will I ever be clear and be able to take a three-month break?" His answer, "No, you have palliative chemo." Not what I was expecting to hear, so yes, lots of tears. Dave looked up palliative chemo for me:

Palliative chemotherapy definition

Palliative chemotherapy is chemotherapy treatment that is given to relieve the symptoms of terminal cancer but not meant to cure cancer or to extend life to a significant degree.

This was a reality check since I am feeling so good. When I arrived at my naturopath's office, I asked to speak to my doctor. He was great and helped to put things in perspective for me. He said my oncologist needs to be very guarded on what he says to his patients, and he is basing it on statistics. He said I do not fit in that box of statistics. He said I am different from other cancer patients; I work harder, exercise harder, eat healthier and live better than most Stage 4 terminal cancer patients. So, take this time to be upset, then in a couple of days, shake it off, and continue to work as hard as you have been. He said he would give me options to "up" my treatment plan by adding more supplements, but we should leave everything until the next CAT scan. He looked at me and said, "Veronica, if something happened to you today, you need to be able to look at the hand you were dealt and know you did everything you possibly could. You should have no regrets because you have done everything you could and more." I thanked him and went off to have the hyperthermia treatment. Still can't quit crying (at the end of the day, I have been working so hard and feeling so good, I just cannot accept I have TERMINAL CANCER). I know tomorrow will be better. I will suck it up and continue to work hard.

July 25, 2019

Yesterday was a tough day. I just finished a break. The time went by so fast. All my chemo side effects were gone. I was working out hard like I used to, feeling really good (normal.) I wished I did not have to go back. A little part of me was hoping I was doing so well I may even get three months' break because I was clear. Also, maybe I no longer needed palliative chemo, and I could have an end date like so many other cancer patients. I get tired of the question—how long will you take chemo for? I say forever, or I stop it. So, I guess this is why after talking to the oncologist and asking him about my scan and also about an end date to chemo, it was like a punch in the stomach. I feel so good. *How can I have Terminal Cancer?* I guess I was just looking for, "Great job, you've got this, and maybe you will be clear at the next scan." But when that did not happen, it was more real.

Just a bad day. I know tomorrow I will have to pick myself up, wipe my tears away, and continue to do what I have been doing.

My morning walks are a form of my meditation. When I am unsure or need an answer, Mom will fly by (red Cardinal) to let me know she is there to support me and to stay strong. I even saw her last night when I went for my walk. She is not ready for me yet. Good news for me. I will try to attach a video that Curtis told me to look at when I was first diagnosed; I listened to it again today. It helps put things back into perspective.

YouTube. Matthew McConaughey, "Life is not easy."

July 28, 2019

Tough weekend. I had such an amazing break; I had forgotten the toll chemo takes on me. It was a tough Wednesday. Then Friday, the nurse came in the morning to disconnect my empty chemo bottle. Feeling not bad after my hyperthermia treatment in Kitchener, Dave took me out for lunch to cheer me up. Lunch was at Stillwater in Paris. It was excellent. We walked around Paris; I was still feeling pretty good. Saturday, I went for my long walk as usual then the nurse came. She set up the anti-nauseous drip after I had a three-hour hydration drip. My older sister Helen dropped by for a visit. It was nice to have the company. I was tired when she left; I think the chemo/ hydration combo had taken a toll on me. I went to bed as soon as she left and woke up at 5:00 p.m, so I missed church (sorry, Mom).

Sunday, when I woke, I was really nauseous (common for me). Even the nurse mentioned I did not look well. She hooked up the anti-nausea drip, then the hydration, and left. I had Dave take the IV pole upstairs for me so I could go back to bed. I slept for three more hours till she came back to disconnect. I sat outside for a while. I had zero energy and felt tired, so I went back upstairs to bed. Slept most of Sunday. I woke up this morning not feeling too bad. The coffee smelt good. I was a little worried I would feel too sick to go to my naturopath, and I might have to cancel. I think sleeping so much Sunday really helped me get better quicker. Bonnie kept texting me: GO TO BED! (thanks, Bonnie). I finally felt well enough today to drive myself to my treatment. I did feel a little queasy, but I made it. I had my vitamin C IV, then drove home. I was starting to feel better on my way home, so I stopped and picked up some groceries, then came home and made us all lunch.

Twenty minutes after lunch, I was sick, unable to keep anything down. I need to remind myself I am still not one hundred percent better. I need to take it easy for another day.

July 30, 2019

Bonnie sent me some beautiful flowers to cheer me up after a rough couple of days. Bonnie has been such a huge support to me. She has learned from her past chemo challenges what works and what does not. Thank you! I, too, want to be sure to help to support others going through cancer. Pay it forward!

August 4, 2019

I hope everyone is having a great long weekend. It has been an amazing week for me. I was better on Tuesday this week and started back to Orangetheory. I was able to get four workouts, and two bike rides in. I will be doing my last ride this morning to end my week. I go for blood work Tuesday, so my port needle will be back in place.

I have more time to do things since I've agreed with the naturopath doctor to decrease my visits. It will be only one vitamin C IV per week and the two hyperthermia on my chemo week. I will see if these changes affect my next CAT scan, which is October 7.

I felt like I bounced back quicker this time (each chemo is different). It was great to be back into a routine. I will continue to go to Orangetheory four times every other week as long as I can. It motivates me to get better sooner. My blood work was great last Tuesday. I will see this Tuesday when I go back for blood work if it remains as good.

August 6, 2019

I ended my week off with a nice forty-eight-kilometre bike ride on Monday. This morning I walked, then off to the hospital to get my blood work done, nervous as always. Hoping all goes well and I can do my chemo. It is 3:30 p.m and still no call, so I am good for tomorrow. Dave and I were just saying how sad it is when you look forward to chemo. I really want to focus hard on getting these last few tumours gone by my next CAT scan.

With that being said, 'He Ho! He Ho! Off to chemo Wednesday I go.'

August 7, 2019

Chemo day was as expected—long and stressful. I arrived at the hospital at 8:30 a.m. I already had my blood work done, so questionnaire, weigh in, see the doctor, take my chemo pills, and start my chemo. I took my pills at 9:00 a.m, saw the doctor at 9:30 a.m. He said I look great. Then he said I look like I am in better shape than him, which was a nice compliment. Off to the chemo room I go. Finally, at 11:00 a.m, I am hooked up with my chemo. I know now it will be after 1:00 p.m before I am finished. Thank goodness this week I was scheduled at 3:00 p.m for hyperthermia. I finally got out at 1:30 p.m, which gave me just enough time to come home, put on some different shorts, have my coffee and leave. My hyperthermia treatment was running behind, too. I did not get started until 3:25 p.m. It would be 4:30 p.m before I was finished. I knew we would be home after 5:30 p.m, depending on the traffic.

As always, my stomach was never good on my chemo days, so another quiet car trip. I try to sleep if I can. When I finally arrived home, I felt exhausted and weak, so I decided to lie on the couch. My stomach started to feel sick, so I took my pills and went to bed early. No chemo voice yet.

August 9, 2019

So far, so good, My sexy chemo voice is back. This morning my coffee tasted good; I am having a second cup now. I went for my walk; then the nurse came to disconnect me. Off to hyperthermia and my IV. I slept through most of my treatment which is good. Today, I even forgot to take the cannabis spray before I got there. I was unsure how the treatment would go, again just a little discomfort the last ten minutes. Dave and I stopped for lunch on the way home at a restaurant in Kitchener, Borealis Grille and Bar. The food was excellent!!

I am still feeling pretty good, so I decided to go for another walk. I know that the next two days may not be as good. Until then, I will take advantage of how I feel.

August 12, 2019

My chemo weekend is over, hurray! But I am still not one hundred percent and have a weak stomach. This weekend I tried to rest as much as possible to see if I would be better quicker. Saturday, I walked before the nurse arrived. I did not feel too bad during the day. I slept off and on and was able to go to church. When I got home from church, I went straight to bed for the night. I was hoping Sunday might not be as bad. But Sunday was a whole new story; I was bad. I felt so weak and shaky when I got up. I knew I was dehydrated. I tried to drink water, coffee, and Gatorade, but nothing was going down well. I took anti-nausea pills and waited for the nurse to hook up my hydration. Once she left, I lay down. I slept most of Sunday. I did not even go outside, which is so unlike me. It is awful; I cannot drink anything, even though I know I need to, I cannot. This week I have more side effects from the chemo. My gums are sore when I brush my teeth or try and eat. Eating soft things is better right now. I went to bed early again in hopes I would feel better tomorrow.

Monday woke up with a huge headache, and my stomach is woozy today. I did go for a little walk, but I had to work up to it. Still feeling weak from the weekend. I drank some Gatorade, which helped. I pray as the day goes on, I get better. Hopefully, tomorrow I will start to be back to normal.

August 13, 2019

I woke up this morning at 6:00 a.m feeling much better. The coffee is still not great, but I can live with that. Two of the side effects of this chemo are my tongue is numb, and I have sore gums. I am back to rinsing with baking soda, which helps relieve the pain. I remind myself I will have to watch what I am eating.

Wow! What a difference a day makes. Yesterday, I could hardly do anything. I napped and sat on the couch most of the day. I was talking to Dave, saying I couldn't believe I had no energy. Today is a totally different day. I looked at my next seven days as holidays, and I plan to enjoy every minute because I know what is coming.

Today I felt so good! I did my six-kilometre walk before leaving for my vitamin C IV (magic juice). The doctor wanted to know my plans for the week since it was my non-chemo week. I told him I was participating in

Orangetheory and my cycling. I shared my details with him, and he smiled and said, "You really love it, don't you?" I'm so glad he gets it.

I received a text from my niece telling me about a cancer ride in London on September 14. So we both signed up for the sixty-kilometre ride.

I went to Orangetheory tonight. It was awesome. It was tough, but I was so glad I went. I am feeling grateful to be able to workout hard again. It gives me something to look forward to when I am on my chemo.

August 15, 2019

With all of the changes I have gone through in the past year with my body and my spirituality, I felt it was time for another Reiki session. My last session was in November, so it was time. Melissa (Reiki Master) has such an amazing way to promote the Reiki session's healing that when it is over, I feel much lighter and more at peace with everything that is happening to my body. I thank Melissa because thanks to her, I am now welcoming my treatments, knowing they will help me cure this disease. Before, I was unhappy with the treatments. Trust me; I do not want to give the impression I like my chemo treatments. I do realize my body needs the chemo and hyperthermia treatments to heal. I understand now this is the journey God wanted me on. Now I am becoming a better person because of this cancer journey. I have learned to live more in the present and not stress about things I cannot control. I have become much more spiritual and feel much closer to my mom.

August 16, 2019

The staff at Orangetheory asked me to be in their promotional video. This is exciting news. They asked me to speak as a cancer patient working out at Orangetheory. The owners spoke to me before the interview and said they had no idea I had Stage 4 cancer because I look so healthy. That is why I love going to Orangetheory so much. The workouts are amazing. We are all working hard. No one knows I have cancer. It feels great to be "normal."

I have been doing a lot of reading and working out as it is so good for your body when you have cancer. Exercise boosts your body's production of T cells, and that improves your immune function. When you exercise, you send signals to your body to get healthier and stronger. Increased blood circulation provides more oxygen and nutrients to your cells, and increased lymphatic circulation carries more toxins and metabolic waste away. Increased circulation also speeds up the healing process. This reinforces my passion for being very active on the days I can.

August 19, 2019

These last few months have been amazing, working out at Orangetheory, cycling, and walking. It has helped me both physically and mentally. I am feeling so good right now; I feel like I am finally getting back into shape. Before I was diagnosed with cancer, my neighbours used to call me 'The Machine.' I was either cycling, running, or swimming. I was always working out. Then came the diagnosis in 2018. I walked, but I was not in shape like I am now. This past year has taught me so much about my life goals, my spiritual goals, and now my exercising/training goals. I feel like I am training for this huge race on October 7 (my next CAT scan). I am trying to eat right, take all the supplements that have been recommended, and then some. My workout schedule is to train as hard as I am able on my good days. I want to ensure my body is in the best shape it has ever been. It is like this is the last hurdle to get over.

So this morning I did a forty-five kilometre bike ride, then came home to a great breakfast Dave made.

After breakfast, I pulled out the angel therapy cards Curtis gave me. I pulled the Archangel Raphael card: 'The healing angel is with you, supporting your healing work.' I am reminded things are as they are meant to be.

August 21, 2019

Today was chemo day. I saw the doctor; My oncologist handed me my blood work said it was great. He said I looked great; go ahead, take your pills, then you can start your chemo. I was hooked up shortly after 10:00 a.m. I saw Gary today. I started with him, and then in February, they switched his chemo days to Tuesday. He has had a rough time, so I was really glad to see him. I saw my uncle Art, too. Dave's cousin was also there; she got a two-month chemo pass because of her CAT scan. I want that!

Also, I saw Sherri. She is another cancer patient I met. She was having her CAT scan and MRI. She is also on a break now, leaving for a trip to the Maritimes Provinces on September 8. Chemo went without a hitch—whew! I set off for hyperthermia. I gave my naturopath a copy of my blood work; he, too, said it was great. So I am certain exercising is helping me to achieve better blood results. I told him that for this chemo, I am doing the water fast only. I was doing 300-400 calories, but I read that water fasting is better. He said he would send me more information on it and the fasting should be started two days before chemo for better results. That will be tough for me because I am still working out. Not feeling too bad when I got home, I went for a walk.

Fasting Information that I read: From Oncology of Nursing News

Why the emerging interest in fasting? In findings from several animal studies, fasting appeared to both reduce toxicity and increase the efficacy of chemotherapy. It also may increase the efficacy of targeted kinase inhibitors (TKIs), although its effect on TKI-related adverse effects is still being studied. The key to the protective factor observed in fasting mice may be a genetic signaling pathway called PKA/EGR1. It appears that when normal cells are deprived of nutrients, they are protected from chemotherapy while dividing cancer cells expend energy while "starving" and are then more susceptible to "attack" by chemotherapy. Also, fasting reduces protein kinase A (PKA) activation and increases AMP-activated protein kinase (AMPK) activity. These signal transduction changes and cause the activation of the early growth response protein 1 (EGR1).

Although animal trials are promising, can the results be translated to patients? In a case report of ten patients being treated for a variety of cancers, those who fasted (water only or with vitamins) for a total of forty-eight to 140 hours before and/or five to fifty-six hours following chemotherapy reported greater tolerance to treatment and less fatigue, weakness, and gastrointestinal symptoms compared with previous nonfasting treatments. Fasting also did not appear to prevent chemotherapy-induced tumor shrinkage or affect tumor markers. Minor complaints during fasting included dizziness, hunger, and headaches at a level that did not interfere with daily activities; weight loss was rapidly recovered.[1]

August 26, 2019

Well, this chemo weekend went a little better than the last one. I did the water fasting this time as it is supposed to help with nausea and other chemo side effects. I think the water fasting this week seemed to help me feel better sooner. Saturday, I had hydration, then went for my walk. I went to church at 5:00 p.m, and when I came home, I went right to bed and slept until 6:00 a.m Sunday.

Sunday was no different. I woke up feeling very sick as usual, had a puffy face and body. The nurse came early, and she gave me the anti-nausea drip and then hydration. I slept for three hours, and when the nurse came back to disconnect, I started to feel much better. She even thought I was beginning to look better. Dave and I went and got some groceries. I could go for a little walk (I am sure I stagger when I walk while having chemo). Still feeling good at supper, I ate. When I woke, I felt okay, a little nauseous, so I took my pills to stay ahead of it.

I think water fasting does help with the side effects of chemo. I only fasted Wednesday and Thursday. Next week, I will start on Tuesday and do three days. Hopefully, this will continue, and I will be able to bounce back quicker.

August 27, 2019

I discussed with my naturopathic doctor my results after doing the water fasting strategy. I told him how quickly I seemed to recover this weekend. He confirmed it was the fasting.

He told me about a study in Turkey with cancer patients fasting during chemo. These cancer patients can take the chemo with fewer side effects and get through the chemo sessions easier. I hope if I continue to fast before and during chemo, I will not struggle so much on my chemo weekends. It's definitely worth a try, and I will continue to monitor the progress.

---

[1] Oncology Nursing News. *Short-Term Fasting Before Chemotherapy in Treating Patients With Cancer.* clinicaltrials.gov/ct2/show/NCT01175837 Updated November 17, 2017. Accessed February 5, 2018.

August 28, 2019

I was back at Orangetheory. When I arrived, they asked me if they could put a story about me in the monthly newsletter. They think it is amazing I come between my chemo treatments and workout. I am humbled they would ask. I think it is important to exercise, to heal your body. It was great to be working out again. I have been waiting all weekend to get back.

I am looking forward to the day that I am rid of this disease so that I can go every week.

September 2, 2019

I always think of my non-chemo weeks as being on a vacation. On those seven to eight days, I do everything I can. I workout each day, walk, pray, meditate and visit with friends. It helps me to stay positive and feel normal. It seems those days go by so fast. This past week I recovered from the chemo quickly, and by Tuesday was back to Orangetheory and worked out each day till Sunday. This morning I did a fifty-kilometre bike ride. Tomorrow it's out to coffee with a friend in the morning, then back to the hospital for blood work and the port being accessed and ready for the next six days.

The side effects from this past chemo were burning throat and heartburn. I struggled to take all of my supplements as swallowing was harder this week. When I did take them, I was sick to my stomach. My fasting will start tomorrow at noon until Friday morning.

September 4, 2019

Wednesday was like every other chemo day—quiet and a little stressful. Due to the long weekend, the nurses are very busy. I am always grateful for their efforts to help me get off to my naturopathic treatments on time.

This week, my stomach is in overdrive, and I am finding fasting is harder to do. I have had headaches, and my stomach is so loud. I push and stay positive that I will hang on until Friday after hyperthermia treatment. I slept through most of it; the last fifteen minutes were painful. My stomach did not feel good on the drive there and back, so it was another quiet ride. When I got home, I went for a walk and felt better.

September 6, 2019

I did it!! I drove myself to my naturopath while on chemo. The nurse came this morning and disconnected me; I still had time for a walk today before I left. I felt good and knew I could do this. While there, I met up with some ladies I have not seen for a while. I feel we are like family. We support each other on the good days and the bad. We hear about each other's CAT scans, chemo sessions, radiation treatments, and surgeries. One of the ladies (Sheila) I have not seen since May, and we shared a big hug. With my changes, I go on different days, so we missed each other. It was so great to see her. She had just finished her radiation, and her cancer has come back. She is moving to Thunder Bay to be closer to her son and daughter. I am so glad I got to see her and share our contact information so we can keep in touch (she passed away in December 2019).

The other lady (Erin) is a young Mom who had breast cancer. She told me today she is cancer-free. Great news and a big hug for everyone. She has a three-year-old daughter. I am so happy for her. Then I got the news about another lady I had not seen in a while. She passed away two weeks ago. She had breast cancer, and it had recently spread to her bones. I saw her in late July after she had undergone radiation for tumours on her spine. It was very aggressive, and the tumours spread to her neck. She had undergone more radiation and then went to the hospice, where she passed away. This loss really upset me. I am reminded to share with everyone that life can change instantly, so enjoy life while you are healthy. 'Never have regrets' is what my doctor always says.

I always say my prayers while lying there and getting my hyperthermia treatment. Today I started to cry. I just keep thinking about the last time I saw her. Trina was telling me that it was getting worse, and they were going to put their house up for sale. It had too many stairs, and with her struggling to walk, this is what they needed to do. That was four weeks ago. Now she is gone. So sad. She was only fifty-one. As I write my journal today, tears come to my eyes.

September 8, 2019

This morning, I woke up not feeling well. I did not feel good when I went to bed and still did not feel good. I had some fresh fruit and waited for the nurse. No coffee. I knew coffee was not going to happen today. The water with cranberry was also not going down well. I wanted to take some anti-nausea pills but struggled to swallow. Even brushing my teeth today was a struggle. The nurse was here at 8:30 a.m. She hooked up to the anti-nausea drip before the hydration. When she left, I lay down on the couch and slept for three hours. I noticed I am feeling a little better. I tried a coffee but dumped it out. I have switched to Gatorade mixed with water. It seems to be going down okay. Once I have a little more energy, I will go for my walk.

I just need to get through today; Monday will be better.

September 8, 2019

Today is our fortieth wedding anniversary. We can't wait to celebrate in November. We have plans to go to Sandals resort in Antigua for a week. This will be after my CAT scan, so we are hoping we have lots to celebrate.

Dave has been my rock and sounding board during this journey. I would not want to be doing this with anyone else. Love you, Dave.

September 9, 2019

I woke up still not feeling one hundred percent. My face was still a bit puffy this morning. I felt ill, lightheaded, and weak. I think I must be dehydrated. I had a bowl of fresh berries, knowing that coffee, juice, or water would not be a good choice. I took some anti-nausea medication to help my stomach. Later in the morning, I felt a bit better, so Dave and I went out and picked up some fresh vegetables. Came home, cleaned them, made spaghetti squash for supper, and Dave made his famous salsa. Later, I went for my daily walk. When I walk, it is my time of meditation. This is when I say my prayers, talk to Mom, Dad, Michael, and Cindy and be thankful for my treatments so I can be healed from this disease.

September 11, 2019

It was great going to my naturopath today. I have not gone on a Wednesday for just a Vitamin C IV since June. We had the same gang on Wednesday. I had been missing them. So I asked when scheduling my September appointments to switch me back to a Wednesday. It was great to see everyone again. The six chairs were full. When I got there, they said how glad they were to see me again. It was good to be back with everyone. It was a quick ninety minutes. When we get together, we talk about everything. It is an information and therapy session all in one. Again, I learned a lot today. Lots of hugs when we were finished.

September 12, 2019

This morning I started back to juicing. We talked about this yesterday at my doctor's. Today I started; I made a 32 oz juice concoction and drank it. It did not take long to make. It was good. I made a vow with myself to do this each morning. The juice had carrots, beets, apples, celery, ginger, and turmeric.

September 14, 2019

My niece Jodie and I accomplished a sixty-kilometre bike ride for the Wheels of Hope. It is a cancer ride from London to Ingersoll and return. It was quite windy going back. I followed Jodie the whole way. You go, girl! We completed the ride in two and a half hours. I am so thankful to Jodie for finding this ride. The money raised helps cancer patients continue to have free rides for their trips to the hospital for treatments.

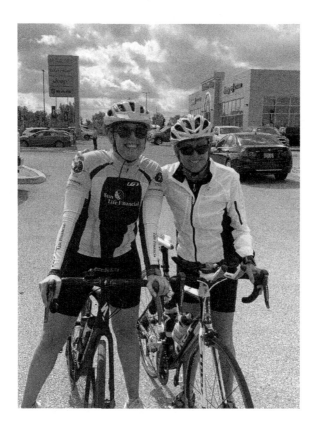

September 15, 2019

It was one year ago today we lost our dad. Whenever I see a blue jay, I think of Dad. He was the strongest and most humble person I have ever known. Miss you, Dad. I know you are so happy up there with Mom and my deceased siblings Michael and Cindy.

September 18, 2019

I went to the hospital on Tuesday to do my blood work to speed things up today. However, it did not work so well. I was the third chemo out and not hooked up until 11:00 a.m. I arrive at the cancer clinic at 8:30 a.m, fill out the questionnaire, get weighed, put my armband on, and wait to see the doctor. My appointment is 9:00 a.m. Since my blood work was good, I take my pills, and now I wait for the chemo. I watch the clock; if I am hooked up by 10:00 a.m, I should be done around lunchtime. Now I am stressed and asking to be finished by 1:00 p.m. I have to be in Kitchener by 2:00 p.m. Chemo days are STRESSFUL! STRESSFUL! The nurse said next time they would "do me first." I honestly would appreciate that and pray it will help to decrease my stress levels!

Today I was out on time and arrived at 2:00 pm. I was able to talk to the naturopath about my food changes and my blood work. I mentioned I have been reading the website 'Chris Beat Cancer.' I listened to a podcast from 'Chris Beat Cancer' about the chemo drug 5FU (the chemo I am taking). In the podcast, he called it 'five feet under,' meaning you will die. So, when I got to this part, I stopped. My chemo and holistic medicine seem to be working for me. Yes, the 5FU may not work for others, but at some point, you need to read but not react. My doctor agreed. He said you need to be careful when you read articles like this as there are no studies to prove what he has done will work with other patients.

We spoke about trying food changes (no meat). He liked the added juicing but was concerned I may not be getting enough protein, and I need to watch and be sure that I am getting my daily requirement. I took notes on his concerns and will be vigilant in making sure I get enough protein.

My blood work was great again this week. I need to keep things going in the right direction. My CAT scan is in October!!!

September 20, 2019

Friday mornings are a good day; I can eat. I have fasted with just water for two and a half days. This morning, I had a slice of zucchini loaf and some fresh fruit with my coffee and chemo pills. The nurse who arrived to disconnect my empty chemo bottle said I looked good today. Friday is the better day of the weekend, but I go downhill after this. It always seems to start Saturday at 6:00 p.m, right after church. I try to stay ahead on my liquids and drink more. I can see the dehydration in the veins of my hands. When I have lots of fluid, my veins are really nice and big. When I am dehydrated, it like those veins have gone missing (that is usually how they are when I go for my vitamin C IV).

I drove myself again this week to Kitchener. I felt okay driving. I did the hyperthermia treatment and my IV. Again, my back aches in the last fifteen to twenty minutes. While I am lying there, I do some deep breathing to alleviate the discomfort. I try not to move much because I do not want the probe on my chest to move. It is over the area where the cancer is. I need the cancer cells to be DEAD. As I lie there, I pray and welcome my treatment will me help fight this disease.

Afterward, I say to myself, 'just suck it up.' It is working to make me better. When the red light finally goes off, I take a deep breath and sit up slowly. I get dressed and am thankful I do not have to do this for another two weeks.

September 23, 2019

This chemo weekend was the same. Not bad on Saturday. Then I started to tank at church. After church, came home and I headed right to bed. I woke up Sunday feeling nauseous as usual. The nurse arrived at 9:00 a.m for the usual routine, and I then, of course, slept on and off most of the day. I went to bed at 6:00 p.m. and slept straight through to 5:30 a.m. Today I am still not well. I am struggling to drink anything. I tried coffee, it did not work, so I tried plain water, then had some fresh berries. They seemed to go down the best. Feeling weak and shaky. I will wait and try to walk later this afternoon.

September 25, 2019

Today is a beautiful Fall morning. I have mentioned before that when I walk, I pray. It is my time to be thankful for my treatments so I can be rid of this disease. I speak to Mom, Dad, Michael, and Cindy and thank them for their love and support.

I wanted to share with you what I have been thinking about the most—my CAT scan. It is on October 7. Yes, Monday after a chemo weekend. If you are a cancer patient or survivor, it is stressful. You hope that everything that you have done since the last scan has paid off.

I have recently changed my eating to mostly vegetables (I have started to add a little meat back into my diet this week because my naturopath doctor was concerned I was not getting enough proteins). I changed to water fasting during chemo treatments. Started to do more intense workouts (Orangetheory). These changes have been positive so far. Will they be enough to help me cross the finish line?

The closer you get to the date, the more you think and pray. Three weeks ago, I went to confession and asked the priest to do the anointing for the sick to me. Bonnie and Jodie (my niece) are at the Vatican in Italy. I asked Bonnie to say a prayer for me. I just wanted to ensure I covered all the bases and to make Mom proud.

September 25, 2019

Today was an IV day in Kitchener, and the topic with the gang there for treatments was CAT Scans. There were a few of us getting our scans done on October 7 and 8. We all talked about how any time we feel something, anything different, we wonder if the cancer has spread. One lady thinks it has spread to another area. She has just started a new chemo pill. She has a pain and thinks that it has spread. We all say we stress before the scan, then stress afterward, waiting for the results. All you want to hear is 'no change' or 'clear.'

I told them that when I think of my CAT scan, I compare it to a final exam or a race. You study or train all semester and hope you have learned enough to ace the exam or do your personal best for the race. You hope the treatments you have been taking are working and hope for positive results. All the ladies laughed and agreed this is exactly what it is like.

October 2, 2019

Chemo day. Coffee does not taste good today. I am hopeful everything goes well at the cancer clinic. I got out at 12:40 p.m, came home, had a coffee, then off to hyperthermia. My back was sore at the end and is still sore. I am hungry, and water and coffee taste awful. I added orange juice to the water.

October 3, 2019

Still struggling to drink. I know I am starting to get dehydrated. I know I need water. My back is sore, and I am hungry.

October 4, 2019

The nurse was here at 8:00 a.m to disconnect me, and then I went for a walk. It is cold out today. When I got home, I cleaned up the kitchen and went out to buy some vegetables. Feels like my colon is full. Made a large bottle of juice. I hope that helps. The chemo pills always constipate me. Still tired, I went to bed early. I have a CAT scan on Monday, so no treatments at the naturopath. You can not have hyperthermia within four to five days of the CAT scan due to the electrodes from the treatment.

October 5, 2019

Feeling a little nauseated. The nurse arrived at 9:00 a.m. Following my routine hook-up and then the disconnect, I went for my daily walk, came home, rested, then got up and went to church. During church, I could feel myself getting sicker. Came home and went right upstairs to bed.

October 6, 2019

Woke up at 4:00 a.m, freezing. Finally got up at 6:30 a.m. The taste in my mouth is so bad. Came downstairs and had some fruit. The fruit seemed to help my stomach. I am still shaky. Coffee seemed good today. The nurse came for my routine of anti-nausea drip and then the hydration. I slept most of the day. I started to feel a little better later during the day and went for my walk. I have my CAT scan tomorrow.

October 7, 2019

When I woke, I was still nauseous. My CAT scan is at noon, so I can drink until 8:00 a.m. But not feeling well, I struggled to drink anything. I went for a walk this morning, trying to kill time and hoping the fresh air will help me feel better.

Curtis drove me to the hospital. I was worried I would not be able to drink the two glasses of liquid, with my stomach feeling so woozy. I was able to get the barium down, though. The nurse came and got me around 12:45 p.m to put the needle in that injects a dye into me, so they get a better picture of the organs. Well, what a surprise! The nurse struggled to find a good vein since I was so dehydrated. She tried three different areas, and finally, one in my forearm worked. This scan never takes long, maybe ten minutes. The hardest thing is the glasses of liquid and the needle. I think I was finished by 1:00 p.m, and Curtis picked me up.

The CAT scans always make me sick, so I knew when I got home, I would be sick. Still not feeling well, I lay down and slept until almost 4:00 p.m. I felt a little better when I got up, definitely still not one hundred percent, though. I know I need to drink, and I will start to get better. It is just so hard to drink when nothing tastes good. I know it will be another early night for me. Hopefully, tomorrow will be a better day.

October 11, 2019

Good morning. Well, the week started slow, but once I began to feel good, I was back doing everything I love to do and feeling amazing. I have been finding with the last few chemo treatments; I am feeling better after lunch Tuesday. Now, Tuesdays are my first class back to Orangetheory. I am always worried about how I will be, so I take my Gatorade for the electrolytes. Once the class starts, I am so into it I forget I have been sick and sleeping for the last four days. Each day I get better. So, this has been a great week. The weather has been amazing. I have had my long walks each morning, then my awesome workouts each night. I will finish my coffee now and go for my walk. Hope everyone has an amazing Thanksgiving. I know I will.

October 16, 2019

The news of my CAT scan results at the cancer clinic was better than planned. I will continue to take chemo. I took a copy of the results to my naturopath, who was very happy with them. I look forward to an updated plan. Today is chemo day. After my treatment is finished, it's off for hyperthermia, then home to sleep for two hours. I will continue to try and sleep away this weekend.

October 21, 2019

This past weekend was a waste of a weekend. I was very nauseous and still not feeling well today. The nurse was here Saturday and Sunday to give me the anti-nausea drip and hydration. I just keep thinking, *you have to get through this weekend.* This is it until after my trip. Dave and I can't wait to go away and celebrate our fortieth anniversary.

October 26, 2019

This week started out a bit slow for my recovery. My stomach still seems to be woozy. My throat is sore—a side effect of the chemo. I started back to juicing and taking my supplements again for the week. I cannot do juicing or supplements while I am doing chemo; my stomach cannot take it. The longer that I am off of chemo, the better my body will become. I am trying to ensure I am back to one hundred percent by November 9 when Dave and I fly to Antigua.

October 30, 2019

I went for my IV today, and while I was there, my doctor and I discussed changes to my plan. He feels if we increase my visit, it will help fight cancer. These changes are aggressive, but we believe it is exactly what we need to see positive results in the January CAT scan. I am in!

Changes and Additions as follows:

Hyperthermia treatments with IV two times a week for two weeks in a row.

Supplements: Deep Immune, Arabinogalactans, Chromium, Vitamin D-K2, Zinc, milk thistle.

I will be administering additional injections of mistletoe to myself two to three times a week (not looking forward to administering this myself but will do it).

Again, this will help to ensure positive results at my next CAT scan in January.

November 6, 2019

Today, I went to my doctor for my last IV before I go away. I also picked up my new supplements, which I will start taking tomorrow. I ordered the mistletoe I will start injecting into myself. I have been off chemo for two weeks now. My sore throat is gone, no more heartburn.

Woo-hoo! Food is tasting much better. I have been juicing and ensuring I am getting all the fruits and vegetables I need. My energy and my sleep pattern are getting better. I will be in great shape when we leave Saturday.

November 8, 2019

Today, I went to the cancer clinic to have my port flushed. They insert the port needle like you were going to give blood, and they flush it with two syringes of saline. They remove the needle, and you are good to go. The flushing is to prevent me from getting blood clots. I have not used my port for three weeks, so it has to be done. I went to 'Goodness Me' to purchase supplements to take with me on my trip, so I don't get sick or have digestive issues.

November 18, 2019

Dave and I had a wonderful vacation. The resort was lovely, the staff was amazing. It was also great to miss the first snowfall and be somewhere warm. Antigua's weather is perfect: thirty-one degrees each day, and it goes down to twenty-five at night. If it rains, it is usually at night or during the day; it is a quick shower. Because of my cancer, my vacation is different. I am much more concerned about what I am eating. I am always trying to ensure I make healthy choices. The resort made great frozen smoothies. You had a choice to make them with either fruits or vegetables or both. I made sure to have one each day. This way, I did not miss the juicing. I was more careful about doing things outside in the sun. I ensured I had 50 SPF sunscreen on, and my port was covered and never exposed to the sun. I tried not to get too much sun. Even going into the ocean or pool is different. I didn't find it as much fun. I guess I am worried I have come so far and do not want anything to set me back. Now it is back to my new normal— treatments, fasting, vitamin C, all starting this week.

November 21, 2019

Yesterday it was back to the grind. Fasting for the next couple of days. IV with hyperthermia. When the IV needle was inserted into my hand, it felt very tender. I figured it would feel better once I lay down for the hyperthermia treatment, but it started to hurt more. The hand is such a tender spot. It was burning when they came in to check on me, and I told them my hand was very sore (I thought about having the needle taken out and put in another spot). They came back with a heated pack, which helped me get through the hour. I got dressed and went to the IV room to finish my IV. Before I left, we went over the new plan and added supplements.

The new changes to my program mean increasing my hyperthermia treatments and added mistletoe injections I will do myself. My naturopath has added more supplements.

November 27, 2019

My blood work continues to be good. It seems what I am doing must be working well. I continue fasting while doing the treatments. Today, the nurse showed me after my hyperthermia treatment how to inject myself with the mistletoe. It does not seem hard, but I will let you know next week when I am on my own. When I return on Friday, she will show me one more time (glad I am a quick study). Giving the needle to myself in my stomach will not be a treat, but it will help kill cancer, so I will do it.

December 3, 2019

I did it today. It was the first day of my mistletoe injections. I did it myself. The nurse gave me a very detailed lesson on how to give myself the injection last week. I was sure I would be able to do it.

She made it simple for me, showed me how to open the vials of mistletoe, fill the needles, and flick it with my finger to get rid of the air bubbles. She showed me how to split my stomach into four quadrants. This way, I am not inserting the needle in the same spot all the time. Each needle must be in a different spot. I need to wipe the area with an alcohol wipe, then gather my skin together, enter the needle just under my skin and inject the mistletoe. I am to do this three times a week. I have got this!

December 8, 2019

Last night, Uncle Gerard passed away. Gerard and his wife Linda have been very supportive of Bonnie and me during our cancer battle. When Bonnie was battling breast cancer in 2017, Linda and Gerard were there for her through her year-long journey. When I was diagnosed in June 2018, Gerard and Linda were there to support me. Gerard was even there to see me at the hospital right after I had my surgery. Last December, Gerard was diagnosed with lung cancer. He has spent this year battling the disease. For the past two months, he struggled as his cancer spread to other parts of his body. Uncle Gerard was a true fighter and will be missed.

December 22, 2019

Dave and I spent a beautiful weekend in Toronto. Walked over to see the Christmas windows at Hudson Bay, then grabbed a cab to the Christmas market, which was very nice. I got my picture taken with a beautiful Christmas angel. We went and had dinner. Then it was off to see 'Come From Away' at the Royal Alexandra Theatre.

December 23, 2019

This morning I went to the cancer clinic to drop off some goodies for the nurses and my doctor. I wanted to hug them and thank them for everything they have done to help me. I will be back on January 7.

While I was there, I dropped off all of the donated goodies I had received from local businesses to go into the cancer bags they give to new patients. I am still collecting items but took what I had. The director of the cancer clinic was so surprised with all that had been donated. These cancer bags will be amazing and uplifting for new cancer patients. It is nice to get little surprises in your cancer bag besides your chemo information. Little things like five-dollar gift cards for Tim Hortons, inspirational notes, ChapStick, free makeup consultation, information on the 'Look Good, Feel Better' program offered through the Cancer Society, socks, gum, and so on. I am so pleased with all the people and businesses that have donated to this great cause.

December 23, 2019

I had opted to go without chemo until January. I chose to do this as my doctor had said I could take a break if CAT scans were good. However, I have to keep in mind that I am on palliative chemo (for life). Before my decision, I discussed my choice with both doctors. My naturopath said,

"I always tell my patients you should never have any regret for your decisions. You should be able to look back and say I did all I could to fight this disease."

He then put a plan together with the following:

He increased the hyperthermia treatments, increased the vitamin C IV, increased the mistletoe by adding mistletoe injections, increased my supplements, and advised me to stick to the Mediterranean diet and continue to fast during treatments.

I have been doing this for the last seven weeks. I am feeling stronger and healthier each day. As the toxins leave my body, most of my chemo side effects are gone, too. I will continue with this plan through January. I also want to update you on how it is going with the self-injections of mistletoe. It's going better than I thought. My hyperthermia treatments are still painful. The treatments have increased. When I pray each morning, I welcome all my treatments knowing that they help me fight this disease.

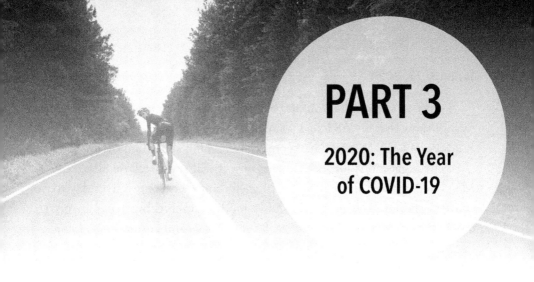

PART 3

2020: The Year of COVID-19

January 10, 2020

I went to the cancer clinic on Tuesday and had my blood work done. I am always so nervous about this. When I got the results later in the afternoon, I was surprised to see that my liver enzymes were high (AST and ALT). Almost double than normal. I have had this a few times before and, with my naturopath's help, have got it back under control.

I called my oncologist to see what I needed to do to get it back down. He was not concerned. He said it has been higher, and we can wait till the end of the month to see what the CAT scan shows.

I also mentioned it to my naturopath when I went for my hyperthermia and IV treatment. I showed him my blood work. Everything else was fine; it was just my liver. He recommended I stop all of my supplements and the mistletoe injections immediately, no Tylenol or alcohol, for one week. Then get my blood work on my liver tested next Wednesday to see if it has gone back down to normal. He believes it is because of the aggressive steps we have taken with all the changes made and supplements that have been added. He cautions me that if it remains high, it could be the cancer.

So now, I wait to see what happens. Next week is an off-week for me, with no treatments. I will get the results the week of January 20. CAT scan will be the following week. This is a reality check for me to slow down and remember I am still not better.

January 21, 2020

I received the results from my bloodwork taken last week on my liver. Results show that my AST had come down 38 but should be <30. Still not at a normal level. My ALT had come down 33 but should be < 36.

New suggestions for supplements now. I will start back on all except MSM and curcumin for now. I will go for another blood test Friday to confirm the levels again. This shows me how everything I put in my body affects it one way or another. I am cautious and ensure I am doing everything I need to do for an excellent CAT scan. I am very nervous. I did not sleep well last night, worrying about my liver status. Now it is 'wait and see' what happens over the next two weeks.

January 27, 2020

Today was the day that I have been waiting for for the last three months. All the hard work I have been doing both at my naturopath and at home—the juicing, eating healthy, injections, hyperthermia treatments, vitamin C IV, working out, meditation—praying all of these changes compare to my heavy-duty training for my marathons, triathlons, or two-hundred-kilometre bike ride. Today is race day. I feel great! I am hoping everything I did will get me across the finish line with success. Thursday, we will see if I did enough.

January 30, 2020

I talked to Dave on the way to the cancer clinic. I told him I think of this as reaching the finish line. Did I do my personal best? Or did I still have some left, and I could have tried harder?

Only my oncologist knew the answer. He was so excited about the results of the CAT scan. He was beaming. He could hardly wait to tell me, "No chemo for the next three months. I will see you after your next scan." I had to hug him and thank him for the wonderful news. He said to go out, see the nurses and hug them, too. Dave and I had a little cry after we got the news. All my hard work had paid off. I did my Personal Best! I texted Curtis to let him know, then called my naturopath. He said he was glad I called him to tell him the great news. Still on a bit of a high, so

Dave is taking me out to dinner tonight to celebrate. Back to fasting for my hyperthermia treatment tomorrow and hopefully a new maintenance plan. Thank you to everyone for all of your prayers!

January 30, 2020

We went to the Cambridge Mill to celebrate. This is where we went for lunch the day before my surgery in June 2018, but now it is for my victory dinner. Our waiter surprised me with 'Congratulations' written on my dessert.

February 6, 2020

A dear friend of mine passed away after a courageous battle with cancer. I met Sherri in April 2019 at the cancer clinic. She was diagnosed with colon cancer. Her daughter is an oncology nurse and often gives me chemo. Her daughter had asked me, when her mother was first diagnosed, to talk to her and her father about my naturopathic treatments. We clicked right away. We would text every week to see how the other was doing. I gave her my naturopath's card. She became his patient, too. Last Thursday, when I got my good news, I texted her but did not receive any response (I wondered if something was wrong). Her daughter texted me Monday to tell me she was in palliative care. I went right to the palliative care unit to see her. I was so surprised since I thought she was doing so well. She had taken a turn for the worst on the weekend. I stayed at the hospital till after 8:00 p.m Monday night. She passed away Tuesday morning. This hit me hard. It just showed me how fragile life is and how it can change in an instant. Sherri was very special and will be missed. I told her I would dedicate my ride for cancer in her honour. I am still in shock. This is why the doctors say celebrate each milestone. You should live for today.

February 27, 2020

I am still going to my naturopath twice a week for IV and hyperthermia, also fasting on those days. I continue to struggle with my back during hyperthermia treatments. I wish I did not have to do them. I am also struggling with my IV, never sure if they will find a good vein. I have been doing this so often for so long. We use both arms and hands. Starting to run out of veins. I will have to start using my port.

I continue to go to the hospital for my blood work and port flush. I am feeling good and doing a lot of walking and spinning on my bike downstairs.

March 6, 2020

I am sure that all of you saw Alex Trebek talk this week about his first anniversary with Stage 4 pancreatic cancer. I listened to him talk about the highs and lows with his continuous fight. When he spoke about the times he wished it was over, I could relate. He talked about his great support. Listening to Alex speak really hit home. You see, I, too, had many times when I was going through my chemo when I felt the same way. I know some people look at me and think my journey has been easy. It has not been. I struggled and continue to struggle just like Alex Trebek (probably like most cancer patients).

My last CAT scan allowed me to be chemo-free for the next three months. **Not cancer-free. Just chemo-free**. When you have Stage 4 cancer, you will never be cancer-free. What chemo-free has allowed me to do is eliminate the chemo from my schedule. All the other treatments continue and have actually increased.

"Covid Alert"

March 13, 2020

Cancelled all Orangetheory classes due to a COVID-19 virus. I am okay with staying at home. Working out at home and walking/running early will be the safest for me at this time. Grocery stores are crazy. People panicked about this virus and hoarded food. Lots on TV about the virus. It is a little scary right now. They have cancelled all flights, and schools and businesses are closed. Only essential businesses remain open with reduced hours. No sports. It is so quiet when you are out walking. It is eerie.

March 14, 2020

The world seems to be going crazy with this COVID-19 virus. I ran today and did my workout downstairs. I am still able to go to church. This would be the last day at church.

March 16, 2020

The world is still crazy with the COVID-19. I am just starting to get a head cold which seems to be getting worst. My appointment with the member of parliament was cancelled due to COVID-19.

I had set up a meeting with our MP to see if the government would look into covering some of the costs for naturopathic treatments. All the naturopathic treatments have been at my expense. I have spent over $90,000 so far, and I am nowhere near finished. I know talking to other cancer patients, both at the cancer clinic and at the naturopath's, they say it is costly but worth it. I know I would not change it for a minute. I believe it should be covered even partially under our Ontario Health Insurance Plan umbrella or through other health care plans. I feel strongly cancer patients or anyone with a terminal disease, where conventional treatments are not enough, should have the option. I was fortunate my co-workers, family, and friends raised money to help with some of the cost. The rest came from my retirement nest egg. I am hoping when our city is no longer in lockdown, we can reschedule this meeting. I believe in this.

Today, I also cancelled my appointment with my naturopath. I am not feeling well, and with COVID-19, it is best to cancel.

March 22, 2020

I had my coffee and daily supplements, then went for a run. It was cooler out, so I ran nine kilometres today. Then I headed downstairs and worked on strength training, showered, and stayed home. Received an email from my naturopath about his clinic letting us know he was considered an 'essential business' and I would be able to continue my treatments. This was good news. I was concerned with me on a chemo break. My naturopathic treatments are the only thing fighting my cancer right now. Getting this news today was very reassuring.

Covid-19 is spreading rapidly every day.

March 25, 2020

Went to my naturopath. Still a little congested. When I got there, there were some changes. The doctor is now wearing a mask. I had to clean and sanitize my hands and answer a COVID questionnaire. Then the doctor was able to start my IV. It took two tries to get a vein in my hand. Hyperthermia treatments continue to hurt the last fifteen minutes. Told him I had just started to get a pain in my abdomen. He told me to call my oncologist when I get home. So I did.

March 26, 2020

I went for walk. Still a little sore today. My hand is bruised from the needle. COVID-19 is crazy. I cleaned and sanitized the house. The hospital called—I go for an ultrasound on my stomach Friday morning. Went for another walk in the afternoon, came home, and watched TV about COVID-19. Started fasting for hyperthermia.

March 27, 2020

I am off to the hospital for an ultrasound on my stomach. Want to see what the pain is. Hopefully, nothing is inflamed. When I arrive at the hospital, things here are now different. A nurse in full hazmat suit met me. I was asked COVID questions, asked to sanitize my hands, and my temperature was taken. After the checks, I was allowed to proceed to the Imaging floor for my ultrasound. The technician mentioned she did not see anything. Good news. I went home, made a coffee, grabbed my purse, and off to my treatment. The nurse set up my IV. The first spot did not work, so tried again in my left hand. It hurt but it worked. Then off to hyperthermia. As I was lying down, my hand was throbbing. If I speed up the IV drip, it hurts more. This hyperthermia treatment and IV was so uncomfortable.

It is scary now with COVID-19. Everything is changing daily, even hourly. All of us need to try and self-isolate as much as possible. For people who have other medical issues, this is a very scary time. I am trying to isolate myself from the public as much as possible. I have been sending Dave out to get groceries and run errands. I am so proud of our Canadian Government—they are doing what they can at all levels to keep us all informed and safe. Thanks to all healthcare workers, fire, police, ambulance, and frontline workers at the grocery stores and drugstores. Thanks to all the people still going to work to keep us all supplied.

We will get through this. We all need to stay safe. Wash your hands often, wear a mask, stay six feet apart when possible.

March 30, 2020

My birthday. Curtis sent me a beautiful text. He wanted to be the first one. I do not have much energy. May lie down for a nap. Due to COVID, I walk early when no one else is walking.

April 6, 2020

I went to the hospital to get my port flushed and blood work only. Still on my chemo break. At the hospital, we needed to practice social distancing. There was a lineup to get in. A nurse meets us with a hazmat suit on. We are asked questions, get our temperature taken, get given a mask, and asked to sanitize our hands. We are even asked why we were there. Then I was off to the cancer clinic. The cancer clinic had also changed. There are not as many chairs in the chemo suite. There were fourteen; now there are six chairs. Your blood work is done in the area that used to be the waiting room. There are a few chairs spread out and where they do the blood work has glass on both sides. The reception where you check-in is all glass now. The hospital seems much cleaner. I went straight home when I was done.

April 8, 2020

Went for vitamin C IV. When I arrived, there were new COVID-19 procedures there also—you sterilize your hands, put on a mask, then off to the IV room. Here too, only one person per room for IV due to social distancing. Our chatty therapy sessions are done. We now text to see who is there. The naturopath has to minimize the patients he has now. The IV took one and a half hours. I read while I was having my IV. Still not having chemo, just having the treatments at my naturopath. I am feeling stronger and healthier every day. I am running more, work out with weights more. Loving it.

April 30, 2020

Today is my CAT scan. I will drink the magic juice. Due to COVID-19, they will use my port for this scan instead of a needle in my arm. This way, they can also flush my port. Since I am not using my port as often, my port needs to be flushed with saline monthly to eliminate the chances of blood clots. It has been longer with COVID restrictions. Using my port was good news since right now, we are struggling to find veins in my arms or hands. When I was ready for my CAT scan, a nurse from the cancer clinic accessed my port. I hope everything is good. The scan does not take long, and I am done. The nurse comes back, disconnects the port needle, and I am good to go. My stomach is so loud it is just gurgling after the scan. I am afraid to go for a walk.

May 6, 2020

I was anxious about my results. I have not had chemo since November. With COVID, my blood work has not been done monthly. I just want to make sure everything is still good. So I called and left a message for my oncologist to see if he could call me later today and give me my results. Then I went for a walk, said my prayers, came home, and showered off for naturopathic treatments. I arrived an hour early for my appointment. Due to COVID-19, you cannot sit in the office if you are early; you must stay in your car until it is your time. No more waiting rooms.

My oncologist called just before 5:00 p.m to give me my CAT scan results. He told me my CAT scan was amazing. I will continue on another three-month break from chemo (yeah!). He said I was in uncharted territory. No other Stage 4 cancer patient with my diagnosis has done this well. Gratitude felt. Enjoy the break. We talked about going back to work; he did not recommend it at this time. He said to continue with my naturopathic treatments as they seem to be working well. I sent a copy of the scan to my naturopath doctor. He, too, was very happy. I had wine to celebrate at supper.

May 10, 2020

Mother's Day. I had my morning coffee, then off for a run. Dave went and picked up flowers for us to take to the graveyard for both of our moms. I feel pretty good today. Curtis came over for supper and gave me a beautiful card. He is my rock. He gets me the most amazing cards. I love him so much.

May 11, 2020

It was snowing this morning. I am off to receive my IV and my consultation with my naturopathic doctor about my CAT scan results. He said I was doing very well; the treatments and the supplements were helping. He said I was doing well because I work hard at it. He said most people, when they start to hear no more chemo or the cancer is gone, take the foot off the gas. It is very important not to do that. We need to ensure we continue to work hard to keep the cancer from coming back.

So I plan to continue with:

Week # 1- hyperthermia and vitamin C IV – Wednesday and Friday.

Week #2- vitamin C IV.

Week # 3 no treatments in the third week.

This would be one IV less per month until the next CAT scan.

When we got home Dave received a message, Dave's dad tested positive for COVID-19. He has been in and out of the hospital a lot since the beginning of this year. Dave is scared since he was with his dad not too long ago. He will need to go and get tested. This upsets me. I cannot risk getting COVID-19.

May 14, 2020

Dave went to get tested for COVID-19. When he came home, he said we can go nowhere until he gets his results. I do not believe he is positive.

May 16, 2020

Today is Dad's birthday. He would have been eighty-two years old. I miss him, but I know he can help me more from where he is.

May 17, 2020

Dave got his results back from the hospital—the test was negative.

May 29, 2020

I have an early appointment today at my naturopath at 8:15 a.m. He started the IV in my hand; it was not dripping, so he had to pull the needle out a bit, then the IV started to drip. My hand is sore. I am hungry and pissed. We go to the hyperthermia room, and he sets it up. I lie down and get ready, my hand is throbbing, and the IV is not dripping steadily. I keep my hand in a fist to try to keep the IV drip going. I can't get comfortable.

My hand is still throbbing. I think to myself I will not make it through the hour. The nurse came in to check on me. I tell her my hand is throbbing and ask if she can remove the IV and try another vein. She moves it from my left hand to my right forearm. It is still uncomfortable, but it is dripping. I try and get comfortable and sleep. I pray to welcome this treatment. I sleep on and off. When the hour is up, I move to another office to finish my IV. It takes another twenty minutes. I leave and drink my shake on the way home. I am later than expected because of my IV issues. I am crabby, so I will go for a walk. Hopefully, it will take me to my happy place!

Lately, when I arrive for my treatment, my heart rate has been really low— 32-35 bpm (normally 45-50). My blood pressure is also low, so the doctor is giving me a nut bar or a drink before he sets up the IV and hyperthermia. You see, I am still fasting. So I will quit eating at 3:00 p.m; until after my treatment the following day. So my fast can be eighteen to twenty hours before I eat. Yet I am still as active, which puts me on a calorie deficit that is too low. One day my heart rate was 30 bpm, and my blood pressure was also low. If your blood sugar is too low, you will get dizzy. Having something to eat allows the sugar to stabilize and prevents the dizziness.

I will try and have some of my shake before leaving for his office, so I have something in my system. We still continue to struggle to find veins to work—two to three pokes before we get one. I may have to start using my port. When I use my port, the IV drip runs over two hours or longer, compared with my veins at ninety minutes. The port needle used at the naturopath's office is smaller than the one I used to get at the cancer clinic, so the flow is slower. Also, there is an additional cost to use your port. I prefer to use my veins as long as I can.

I have been increasing my cycling. I am training more like before I had cancer. I am making sure to eat really well. I have been doing a lot of cycling and longer distances. My neighbour made the comment, the "Machine is Back" after our ride together. As mentioned earlier, my neighbours called me the 'machine' since I was always training for something—marathon, triathlon, long-distance cycling. Hearing this was a sign I am getting stronger and back to normal.

With COVID-19, as mentioned, I have been unable to get my blood work done each month consistently like I was doing. I keep track of all of my blood work results, so I can see how my body is doing. It is a way for me to check on how I am doing since I am not taking chemo. I need to know what I am doing is still working. I am nervous. The cancer clinic called today and said I would start back in July for blood work. This is great news! They also gave me the date for my next CAT scan—August 11. I am hoping for another really good scan. I have been working so hard to do everything right. I hope it is paying off.

We are now entering into a new phase (orange zone) of COVID-19. More businesses are starting to open. I am still reluctant to go back to Orangetheory, though. I have cancelled my membership. I purchased a rowing machine and step like we used at Orangetheory, allowing me to workout at home. I do not want to put myself at risk of catching COVID-19. Orangetheory was very understanding. They knew how well I was doing and did not want to take the risk. I miss everyone but I know it is for the best. When I did the promotional video for Orangetheory, they emailed it to all of the members in our monthly members' bulletin. After the email was sent, a lot of the members told me they were surprised I had Stage 4 cancer and were amazed I would come and work out the weeks I was not taking chemo.

Wednesday July 1, 2020

Canada Day. We usually have a big family pool party but not this year, due to COVID-19 and social distancing. Instead, I went for an eighty-kilometre bike ride with Jerry. It was an awesome ride.

Saturday, July 4, 2020

Lauren (a newly diagnosed cancer patient) called to talk about cancer. She was given my name by the nurses at the cancer clinic. She, too, had Stage 4 colon cancer. She was only thirty-one. She wanted to talk about my treatments at my naturopath because she is thinking of going there. We spoke for a while. I have added her to my daily prayers. I am honoured the nurses from the cancer clinic thought I would be a great support person for her. I continued to text her to check in and see how she was doing.

July 8, 2020

I am fasting. I made my shake to have after my treatment. Hyperthermia and IV today. I slept on and off during the treatment. Still uncomfortable. I asked the nurse about Sheila. I had been thinking about her lately. She was the lady I met here, and the last time I saw her, was last September, and she mentioned her cancer was spreading. She had also mentioned she was moving to Thunder Bay to be with her family. She was excited about purchasing a new condo and also being close to her family. I said I had texted her a few times. I didn't receive a text from her last Christmas and have not heard from her since. The nurse told me she died last December. She said she got sick within a month after she moved to Thunder Bay. She never got into her new condo.

July 9, 2020

I received a text from JD. She is a lady I have seen every Wednesday at my naturopath's office. She goes there for IV treatments and has Stage 4 lung cancer. Her CAT scan results were not that good. She wants to start to take hyperthermia and also do the mistletoe needles. She said I had good results, and she wants to try it. She is worried about the cost.

July 10, 2020

Dave is driving me today to my appointments. I am very hungry today, as usual. We get there, and the nurse sets up my IV. We go to the hyperthermia room, and she sets it up. I lie there and watch the drip. I try to speed up the drip so that it will finish at the same time as my hyperthermia. Then I will not have to wait and go to another room. It does not. Used the vein on my right forearm. My veins are not taking the IV as fast. After my hyperthermia treatment is finished, I go to examination room one to wait for the IV to finish. When done, the nurse will unhook my IV, and I can leave. I am not back for two weeks. When I return, it will be only for an IV treatment.

July 22, 2020

Hospital called. Mammogram and CAT scan both scheduled for August 11.

July 29, 2020

I was not feeling well. I went for a walk, then off to my treatment. The nurse checked my vitals, then set up the IV. We used my left arm. She could not find any really good veins today (surprise), so we used the elbow on my left arm. The vein was very hard to get through, and when it did, it hurt. I had to keep my arm straight. We went to the hyperthermia room and got set up. My arm was sore, but as long as I held it straight, it would drip. The nurse put the probe on my abdomen and a blanket on my shoulders. My feet were freezing. I thought they would get warm, but they didn't. I slept off and on through most of the treatment. The last nineteen minutes were bad. My arm was sore; my back was sore. I was uncomfortable; my feet were cold, and I wanted this treatment over. I was praying to welcome the treatment, but I could not wait for it to be over. When I got home, I received an email from the cancer clinic with my blood work results. Everything looked good except my AST and ALT (liver). They were four times higher.

I called my oncologist, who was not concerned. He said it had been that high before. I sent the blood work to my naturopath. He immediately asked me to stop all supplements except my silymarin and get my blood work done in seven to ten days. Not what I wanted to hear; I am concerned. Since I am not taking chemo, I am not getting my blood work done monthly due to COVID-19. I feel like I have no idea right now how I am doing inside. It makes me very nervous. I am concerned my CAT scan may not be good, either.

July 31, 2020

I did not sleep well. Worried about my liver. Not feeling well today. I went for my walk, made my shake, and got ready to go to my treatments. I got there, and the nurse did my vitals. My blood pressure was 110/60 —that was low for me. My oxygen was 100. But my heart rate was 37 bpm. She redid my vitals four times, then called the doctor. He did not like that my vitals were so low. He gave me a bar and some juice. I am fasting and had nothing to eat. I started to feel a little better. They hooked up the IV and then the hyperthermia. The IV was slow. I finally get my blood work done next week. I am hoping my liver enzymes will be back to normal. My doctor is not concerned. Cancer clinic called—they will start doing monthly port flushing and blood work again (yes!). It was cancelled due to COVID-19. This is great news. I track all of my blood work results; I compare week to week. My oncologist thinks my CAT scan will be amazing and thinks I can go back to work on a modified work-from-home plan. I hope so.

August 3, 2020

While I was at my naturopath's, I learned that Lauren is not doing well and has cancelled all her appointments. It might be why she has not returned any of my texts. I was texting weekly to see how she was doing.

I also learned Angela had just finished radiation on her neck. The results were not good. Her oncologist gave her some chemo pills and said this is all they can do for her (not what you want to hear). It seems like every six months, I lose someone I have met during my cancer journey. She was a regular Wednesday IV groupie. This scares me, and it really hits home. You can be doing well; then cancer comes back with a vengeance.

August 10, 2020

I finally received a text from Lauren. She has been struggling with fluid in her stomach, and they don't know why. She is getting her stomach drained. She told me she is having a CAT scan on Wednesday. I told her mine is tomorrow. We promised we would text each other with our results.

August 11, 2020

Today is my CAT scan and mammogram. I am not eating. I have to be at the hospital at 7:30 a.m. At the hospital, I registered for my mammogram. It was done and then off to get my CAT scan, which was done by 9:20 a.m. Now, I wait for my results!

August 14, 2020

The nurse texted me from my naturopath. She sent me Angela's obituary. This had been her third bout of cancer (thirteen years of fighting). She really struggled this time. She will be greatly missed and was a very special lady. She was a Reiki Master. She also was a dog walker for the animal shelter. She would do Reiki sessions for cancer patients, and she helped JD. She was a regular in our Wednesday IV group. She was the one who got me on the juicing, and other cancer-fighting foods. She was a part of my Cancer Family.

August 25, 2020

Today, I was finally able to meet with the MP to discuss the possibilities of the government adding to our Health Care coverage some costs for naturopathic treatments. I focused on cancer patients. The meeting was good and promising. Then I went to the cancer clinic for my blood work and received my CAT scan results.

My blood work was good. My liver enzymes are still high but coming down. My CAT scan results were excellent. The spots on my lungs are unchanged, and my colon, omentum, lymph nodes, and liver show no signs of cancer. Yes!!! I am now able to start back to work. It will be a transitional back-to-work program. I will be working from home. I am nervous but excited. I am ready. I called work to let them know. Today was a big day—a start of going back to Normal Life.

I texted Lauren to let her know my results. She, too, was to get her results and would let me know. I did not hear back from Lauren. I hope everything is okay.

August 29, 2020

Today was the Virtual Conquer Cancer Bike Ride. Due to COVID-19 restrictions, the event was virtual.

I registered last year when I was there cheering on my niece and my neighbour. While waiting, Dave and I went to the registration tent, and I signed up as a *cancer survivor*. It is my goal to ride again. This time I said I would be riding as a cancer survivor and would ride with the yellow flag. I did it. I rode eighty kilometres with the yellow flag—a cancer survivor.

My friend Jerry, my neighbour and I all rode eighty kilometres. Later that night, my neighbour and her husband came over to celebrate my cancer victory with a glass of wine.

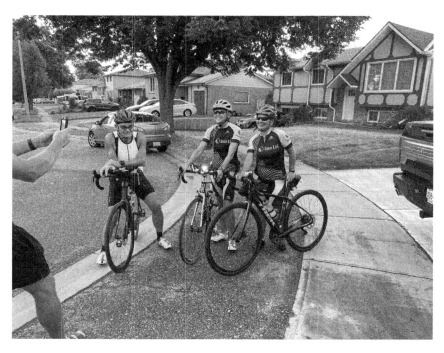

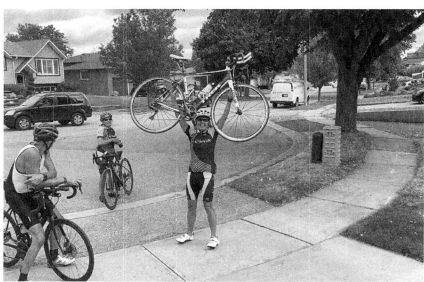

August 31, 2020

I had to go back for another mammogram and ultrasound. The left breast had changed, and they just wanted to be sure. If I do not hear within a week, everything is good.

September 8, 2020

Today is our forty-first wedding anniversary. It is hard to believe that two years ago, we were crying and unsure how many more we would have. This year, I told him he is stuck with me for a while yet.

In a few weeks, I will be going back to work. I will work remotely, and it will be a gradual progression. I am frightened to go back. I do not want stress. I want to help others, pay it forward and do something I really want to do.

September 9, 2020

I got the news today that Lauren passed away. She was diagnosed recently. This one upsets me. She was so young; she had three children. The youngest will be a year old in October. Even though I had never met her, she was another one in my Cancer Family. I prayed for her daily, hoping she would recover. It makes me wonder why I am still here. What am I doing differently? How long will it last?

September 15, 2020

I received a text from a friend of mine, Mike, who had just been diagnosed with prostate cancer. He was also going to my naturopath. Once he was diagnosed, and due to the COVID-19 restrictions, he decided to do naturopathic treatments while waiting for surgery. He was hoping for good results like me. As a new patient, you need to get blood work done before the vitamin C IV. While he was at a clinic in Kitchener giving blood, he talked to the nurse about me and my diagnosis. A lady in another room overheard the conversation, and she, too, had been diagnosed with Stage 4 colon cancer. She apologized for eavesdropping but was so intrigued with the story since she had just started as a new patient at my naturopath and was there getting blood work. She asked if he would give her my number to call and talk to me. So Mike texts me to get my approval.

September 23, 2020

I went to see my family physician. One of my veins has remained swollen long after an IV treatment. The vein is in the under part of my forearm, so I am constantly irritating it, and now it is protruding and very tender. It has been like this for two months. It does not seem to be getting better, so I wanted the doctor to look at it.

At first glance, my doctor thought it could be a blood clot and sent me for an ultrasound.

The results showed there was no blood clot, but the vein was inflamed due to the IV. He said it could be months before it will go back to normal.

September 28, 2020

I started back to work today. I am working remotely from home with a gradual progression back to full-time. My employer has been so good to me during this journey. They had fundraisers for me to help cover some of the cost of my naturopathic treatments. I have to thank my boss for always keeping in touch with me and believing I would be back. When I got my diagnosis, I never thought I would be back. My boss continued supporting me and telling me I would have a job to come back to. I have nothing but gratitude for him. Yes, I am excited to be back, but I am scared. I have spent the last two and a half years going to treatments, and now I was back to work with minimal naturopathic treatments and CAT scans. My boss has promised they would work around my treatment schedule. They were just glad to see me back!

My next CAT scan is on November 26. Hopefully, my health will be the same.

September 30, 2020

I went for my hyperthermia treatment. Again my heart rate was low, so I had to have something to eat before the treatment.

When I got the ultrasound results from my family physician, I emailed my naturopath to see if I could eliminate my extra IV. I will keep the IV with my hyperthermia treatments. I was hoping I could have a break. I haven't had one yet this year. My veins need a break. He has agreed a break would be good for me. He also suggested I start using my port.

October 5, 2020

I received a call from a lady named Penny who has just started treatments at the same naturopath I go to. She had heard about my story from my friend Mike who was also now doing treatments there. Penny wanted to know everything about my surgery, all my treatments, and the chemo I was on, how long I had been taking chemo and so on. After I told her my story, I asked about her. She was fifty-one, diagnosed in 2017, and was on the chemo pill. She has tried all the other chemo options, and nothing is working. This chemo pill was her oncologist's last method of treatment for her. This is why she was now doing hyperthermia. She is finding it very costly to continue with this. She told me she had to sell her car to cover the payments. It breaks my heart. Why should a terminal cancer patient have to sell things to afford treatments? After I hung up, I decided it was time to start sending out letters to other people in the government who I think could help with the costs.

October 9, 2020

My niece Melissa (my Reiki Master) completed all of her breast cancer treatments. She was able to ring the bell today. She was diagnosed at the end of last year. Luckily, she was able to get her surgery completed before COVID-19 closed all surgeries. Congratulations!! I am so proud of her.

October 12, 2020

Thanksgiving morning. As I walk, I can hardly believe I am cancer-free and back at work. Who would have thought two and a half years ago, when I was diagnosed, this would even be possible? Last month Dave and I celebrated our forty-first wedding anniversary. Two years ago, there were a lot of tears, and we were not sure how long I had. This is amazing. Lots to be thankful for! Let's see what the next CAT scan shows in November. I want to hear the oncologist tell me, "I am cancer-free."

October 21, 2020

I left for my treatments. I had hyperthermia and IV and then came home. It was raining. I worked more then went for a walk. Still hurts to sit. I talked to Penny again while I was walking. She is starting to flip out. Her blood results were not very good. Her CEA cancer marker numbers were two times higher. She was taking new treatments at the naturopath, and her oncologist had also started her on a new pill. I felt so bad; I tried to reassure her things would be okay. She has recently made a lot of changes, with new chemo addition of hyperthermia and vitamin C. So this may have caused the spike. I told her to try and stay positive and trust what she is doing now will help. I asked her to call her oncologist and ask him and see what he recommends. You have to trust the system. These doctors are familiar with this. She said she would call him. I was thankful she had called me and was feeling better after we had talked.

CEA blood test for cancer patients is a vital test. It lets us know where we are. You want to be less than five. The higher the number, the more cancer cells you have in your body.

October 31, 2020

I did not sleep well again. I am doing a lot of tossing and turning. My butt muscles are sore. I walked this morning; my feet and hands were freezing when I got home. I emailed the Naturopathic Cancer Cost letter to our Member of Parliament, Christine Elliott, today. Hopefully, it will go somewhere. It breaks my heart to know a Stage 4 cancer patient is worried about paying for treatments. So right now, I need to be the voice.

November 13, 2020

I got up, went for a walk, then off to my treatments. I got there a few minutes early and was hooked up. Both days this week, I was hooked up early and was finished by 11:00 a.m. Then, I went for another walk. I sent emails about my naturopathic treatment costs to Ontario Cancer.org, and the Canadian Cancer Society. Not sure I will get anywhere.

November 21, 2020

Whenever I walk now and see a dog, I think about how much I miss having a dog. When I was going through all my treatments, we never had time to think about a dog. Today, Dave and I went and looked at German shepherd puppies. We have had three German shepherd dogs. Our last dog Tika was the best. Now things are semi back to normal, and my treatments have slowed down, so we figured it was time to add a new puppy. We bought one. She is amazing.

November 26, 2020

I had my CAT scan today. They tried my port three times, then had to use my arm. When I was done with the scan, I had to stop off at the cancer clinic so they could look at my port. It worked fine. I was told by my family physician I would need a colonoscopy and set up an appointment.

Today I went to see the surgeon for a colonoscopy. He said that I looked terrific and had been through a lot. Looking at my charts, he said when patients are Stage 4, they do not do a colonoscopy. He said most patients are so far gone a colonoscopy would be of no value. He was really good. He mentioned I was not the 'normal' Stage 4 cancer patient. He said you are doing AMAZING; keep it up.

December 2, 2020

I am off for my treatments. The treatment went fine until the last fifteen minutes. Dave drove, which was a nice change. I went for a walk but no workout because I was feeling a little tired.

December 3, 2020

I worked today. It was busy. I was able to go for my run before work and able to walk Piper (my new puppy). I worked till 3:30 p.m, which makes a long day. My oncologist called with my CAT scan results. He said, "I was cancer-free." I have been waiting to hear those words. I replied, "Like I am in remission?" He responded, "Yes." Great news. Finally. I have crossed the finish line!!!!! I am finally cancer-free. My oncologist said the two words—CANCER-FREE—that I had been waiting to hear. He also reviewed my blood work and my CEA results. I was less than two. He mentioned I should celebrate and asked if I wanted to move out the CAT scans to every four months. I agreed to both. Because of COVID-19, Dave and I had a glass of wine to celebrate since we still cannot go out!.

December 4, 2020

I went for my treatments today and could not wait to share my news with my naturopathic doctor. The clinic was thirty minutes behind schedule, so today, I could finish the hyperthermia and IV simultaneously. We went over the results of my CAT scan, and my naturopath thought they were excellent. He said not many people with your diagnosis have done as well. Not Stage 4 cancer. What we do going forward will be new to both of us. He said you are now writing your own playbook for Stage 4 cancer. Then we discussed what to do for the next four months' treatments.

We will change the treatment schedule to two hyperthermia and vitamin C IV a month, plus the injections I do and my daily supplements. Yeah! We will review the plan after the next CAT scan, which is April 6, 2021.

My race is not over yet. I will continue to train as hard. I will continue to do everything possible to keep this disease out of my body. My CAT scans will continue for the next year every four months.

What do I think made the difference in my diagnosis?

From the beginning, I treated this diagnosis like training for a race, I would do whatever it took to get my personal best (get rid of this disease). There is some training you do not want to do, but you do it because it will make a difference in the end.

Also, following the guidance of my medical team and doing both conventional chemo with the naturopathic treatments.

My biggest motivating factor? Faith, daily prayers. Mostly, just knowing Mom, Dad, Michael, and Cindy were watching over me!

ACKNOWLEDGEMENTS

Thanks to my medical team at both the cancer clinic and naturopathic clinic. Thanks to the nurses who treated me at my home on chemo weekends. Thanks for the love and support from all of my family and friends.

A special thanks to my parents, who taught me early how to be strong. They showed me no matter how hard things are, you keep going.

Every day I thank God for another day and for helping me welcome all my treatments so I can stay healthy and free from this disease.

Thank you for following my journey.

TERMINOLOGY

CAT (or CT) Scan

You lie in a tunnel-like machine while the inside of the machine rotates and takes a series of X-rays from different angles. These pictures are then sent to a computer, where they're combined to create images of slices, or cross-sections, of the body.

Doctors order CAT scans for a long list of reasons:

CAT scans can detect bone and joint problems, like complex bone fractures and tumours. If you have a condition like cancer, heart disease, emphysema, or liver masses, CAT scans can spot it or help doctors see any changes. They show internal injuries and bleeding, such as those caused by a car accident. They can help locate a tumour, blood clot, excess fluid, or infection. Doctors use them to guide treatment plans and procedures, such as biopsies, surgeries, and radiation therapy. Doctors can compare CAT scans to find out if specific treatments are working. For example, scans of a tumour over time can show whether your body is responding to the chemo or radiation in a manner it was intended.

Chemo Port

A chemo port is a small, implant reservoir with a thin silicone tube attached to a vein. The main advantage of this vein-access device is that chemotherapy medications can be delivered directly into the port rather than a vein, eliminating the need for needles. The doctor will make two small incisions—one at the base of your neck and another on your chest

135

about two to three centimeters below your collarbone—then insert the port into the opening on your chest. The doctor then tunnels the catheter under your skin toward the cut at the base of your neck and into your vein. Ports can remain in place for weeks, months, or years. Your team can use a port to: reduce the number of needle sticks and give treatments that last longer than one day. You can swim with your implanted port as long as there is no needle in place. The skin over your implanted port doesn't need any special care. You can wash it as you normally would.

Palliative Chemo

Cancer specialists (oncologists) recommend chemotherapy in one of two situations. For some cancers, chemotherapy can completely get rid of the cancer with a good chance that it will never come back. Examples include certain types of lymphoma, leukemia, and testicular cancer, among others. For most cancers that have metastasized (spread beyond the original cancer site), chemotherapy cannot cure the cancer. However, chemotherapy may help shrink the cancer, improve or eliminate distressing symptoms caused by the cancer for a period of time and help you live longer. The use of chemotherapy in these situations is called palliative chemotherapy.

Loco-Regional Hyperthermia

Loco-regional hyperthermia (LRHT) consists of a table with two electrodes that deliver a controlled energy dose to a localized treatment area based on the concept of capacitive coupling to generate ion flow and heat. Target temperature: 41-45 degrees Celsius. Penetration depth at low frequency allows for the treatment of deep-seated tumours. Treatment length: sixty minutes per treatment.

Vitamin C Mistletoe IVs - Treatment Length 90 mins

Vitamin C is a nutrient found in food and dietary supplements. It is an antioxidant and also plays a key role in making collagen.

High-dose vitamin C may be given by intravenous (IV) infusion (through a vein into the bloodstream) or orally (taken by mouth). When taken by intravenous infusion, vitamin C can reach much higher levels in the blood than when the same amount is taken by mouth.

High-dose vitamin C has been studied as a treatment for patients with cancer since the 1970s. Laboratory studies have shown that high doses of vitamin C may slow the growth and spread of prostate, pancreatic, liver, colon, and other types of cancer cells.

Some laboratory and animal studies have shown that combining vitamin C with anti-cancer therapies may be helpful. In contrast, other studies have shown that certain forms of vitamin C may make chemotherapy less effective.

Animal studies have shown that high-dose vitamin C treatment blocks tumour growth in certain models of pancreatic, liver, prostate, and ovarian cancers, sarcoma, and malignant mesothelioma.

Mistletoe therapy acts on many levels. On the one hand, it boosts the immune system by multiplying and activating immune cells. On the other, mistletoe therapy can induce apoptosis (the process of natural cell death) in tumour cells which results in the inhibition of tumour growth.

Healthy tissue is not adversely affected by this. On the contrary, immune cells and other healthy cells are protected against further injury, e.g., damage caused by cytostatic drugs.

Benefits of potassium and magnesium: it produces energy and regulates blood sugar and chemical reactions in the body. Magnesium helps maintain the proper levels of other minerals such as calcium, potassium, and zinc. Your heart, muscles, and kidneys all need magnesium to work properly. The mineral also helps build teeth and bones.

Benefits of calcium

Your body needs calcium to build and maintain strong bones. Your heart, muscles, and nerves also need calcium to function properly. Some studies suggest that calcium, along with vitamin D, may have benefits beyond bone health: perhaps protecting against cancer, diabetes, and high blood pressure.

Acupuncture

Acupuncture is a type of therapy involving the placement of tiny, hair-thin needles into certain pressure points on the body to relieve various conditions. Acupuncture is one of the oldest forms of traditional Chinese medicine, dating back to at least 100 BCE. While acupuncture is accepted as a form of medicine in many parts of the world, the jury is still out in the West. Nonetheless, millions of people each year find acupuncture provides relief for a surprisingly broad range of symptoms.

Cupping

What is cupping therapy? The suction and negative pressure provided by cupping can loosen muscles, encourage blood flow, and sedate the nervous system (which makes it an excellent treatment for high blood pressure). Cupping is used to relieve back and neck pains, stiff muscles, anxiety, fatigue, migraines, rheumatism, and even cellulite.

Benefits of cupping therapy: people who turn to cupping therapy often do so to improve mobility and ease muscle soreness, pain, and surgery recovery.

"The two biggest reasons cupping is used is to decrease pain and increase your range of motion."

Reiki

Reiki is a form of energy healing that originated in Japan in the early 20th century. According to the *International Center for Reiki Training*, the practice is based on the idea that we all have an unseen "life force energy" flowing through our bodies. A Reiki practitioner gently moves her hands just above or on the client's clothed body, helping reduce stress and promote healing by encouraging a healthy flow of energy.

According to a 2007 survey conducted by the National Institutes of Health, 1.2 million adults and 161,000 children in the United States received energy healing therapy like Reiki in the previous year. A growing number of Americans now use reiki to help with relaxation, anxiety, pain management, and depression, according to a study in the March–April 2017 issue of *Holistic Nursing Practice*.

Supplements

Deep Immune: represents a unique marriage of the Western herbalism approach and the traditional Chinese Materia Medica. Qi tonics are valuable to anyone who wants greater energy, increased resistance to flu, colds, and other infections, and aid the treatment of immune system disorders.

Deep Immune, Cancer and Dr. Neil McKinney, ND

Dr. Neil McKinney has written the influential textbook Naturopathic Oncology. He explains that astragalus-based formulas have shown a high degree of scientific rigour to mitigate the harm done by chemotherapy while improving survival. From his own experience, founded on long years of clinical practice, Dr. McKinney provides a resounding confirmation of the effectiveness and utility of astragalus-based formulae. He asserts that, "It can double the chance of a good response, while reducing side-effects by one-third to one-half. My current favorite formula is Astragalus Combination from St. Francis Herb Farm, also called Deep Immune formula."

Methylsulfonylmethane (MSM)

In terms of cancer healing, methylsulfonylmethane is increasingly being considered as a consistent and proven modality. As a stand-alone, it has been shown to reduce breast cancer tumours. This includes those in triple-negative breast cancer, which often does not respond to conventional forms of cancer treatment. MSM also promoted cancer cell "apoptosis" (or cancer cell death) in certain gastrointestinal and esophageal cancer cell lines, according to a 2012 study published in the *Journal of Gastrointestinal Cancer*.

The specific mechanisms by which MSM does its work on cancer are still being studied. However, many health experts point to its ability to rid the body of lactic acid in the bloodstream (thus changing the environment where cancer cells thrive). They also note its presence as an anti-microbial.

Silymarin: Herbal medicine

An extract of milk thistle (Silybum marianum) seeds, which has been used for hepatitis and cirrhosis, the major constituent of which is silibinins A and B. The active component, silymarin, has antioxidant and hepatoprotective actions. Silymarin helps prevent toxin penetration and stimulates hepatocyte regeneration effects: liver detoxification, improved dyspepsia symptoms, decreased fasting blood glucose.

Metatrol PRO is shown to support healthy cell metabolism in abnormal cells, exhibiting non-oxidative glucose metabolism, increasing Oxygen Consumption Rate (OCR), and reducing production of lactic acid (ECAR). In animals implanted with abnormal cells, Metatrol PRO, at a dose comparable to 41 mg of FWGE-SC per day for a person, controlled cell growth as well as 5,500 mg/day of FWGE. Also, studies of gene expression showed that genes associated with abnormal cells were downregulated and genes associated with healthy cell function were upregulated.

Arabinogalactan: Health Benefits of Arabinogalactan

1) Help Combat Cancer.
2) Improves Immune System.
3) Alleviates Allergies.
4) Helps Combat Pathogens.

Vitamin D3 Benefit #1: Reduces Risk of Cancer

Vitamin D3 decreases cell multiplication and acts as an anti-inflammatory. In recent studies, inflammation is a critical element of tumor proliferation. Numerous studies have presented a link between high vitamin D levels and a lower risk of cancer. In a study called *Health Professionals Follow-up,* subjects were half as likely to be diagnosed with colon cancer with a high concentration of vitamin D3 as those with low levels. Similar findings have shown that Vitamin D3 intake can possibly lower the risk of breast cancer. Although a definitive answer cannot be made at this time, studies are promising that high levels of Vitamin D3 have a link with lower cancer risk.

Summary: Physicians have found that vitamin D if taken for at least three years, could help cancer patients live longer. The findings suggest that the vitamin carries significant benefits other than just contributing to healthy bones.

Zinc

Zinc, a nutrient found throughout the body, helps the immune system and metabolism function. Zinc is also important for wound healing and your sense of taste and smell. With a varied diet, your body usually gets enough zinc. Food sources of zinc include chicken, red meat , and fortified breakfast cereals.

Curcumin

Supplementation of curcumin reliably reduces markers of <u>inflammation</u> and increases the levels of endogenous antioxidants in the body.

REFERENCES

Hay, Louise L. 1987. *You Can Heal Your Life*. Santa Monica, CA: Hay House.

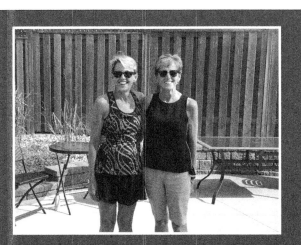
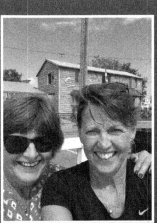
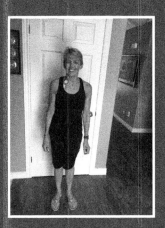
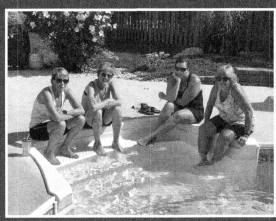

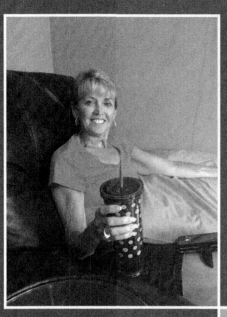
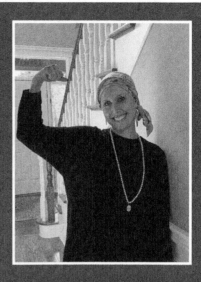
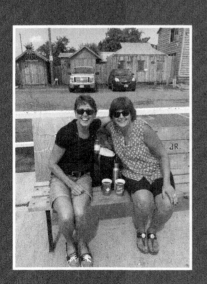
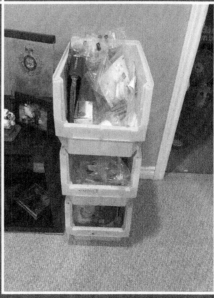

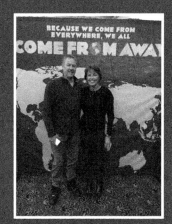
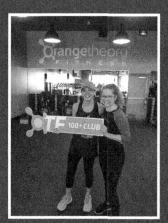
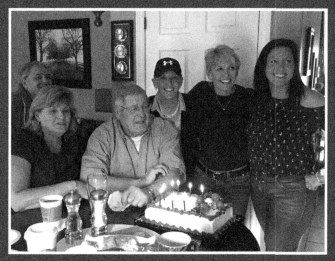
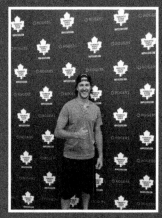
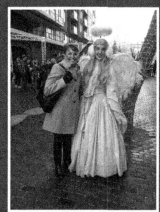

Printed in Great Britain
by Amazon

37911278R00088